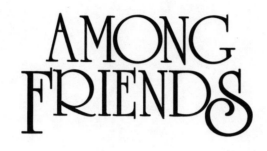

AMONG FRIENDS

AMONG FRIENDS

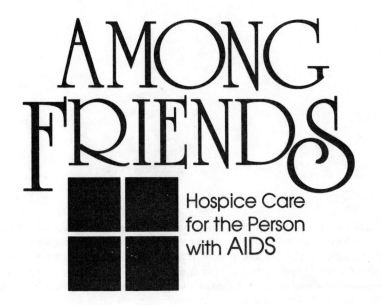

Hospice Care
for the Person
with AIDS

ROBERT W. BUCKINGHAM, Dr. P.H.

Prometheus Books
Buffalo, New York

126391

Published 1992 by Prometheus Books

96 95 94 93 92   5 4 3 2 1

Library of Congress Cataloging-in-Publication Data

Buckingham, Robert W.
    Among friends : hospice care for the person with AIDS / by Robert W. Buckingham, Dr. P.H.
        p.   cm.
    Includes bibliographical references.
    ISBN 0-87975-720-5 (alk. paper : cloth)—ISBN 0-87975-759-0 (alk. paper : pbk.)
    1. AIDS (Disease)—Palliative treatment. 2. Hospice care. I. Title.
    [DNLM: 1. Acquired Immunodeficiency Syndrome. 2. Hospices. WD 308 B923a]
RC607.A26B83   1992
362. 1'969792—dc20
DNLM/DLC
for Library of Congress   91-45568
                                                                          CIP

Printed in the United States of America on acid-free paper.

Dedicated to the spirit and memory of my father

"You can do whatever you set your mind to do."

William R. Buckingham

Contents

Acknowledgments   9

Prologue: Lessons from My Patient-Teachers   11

1. The History of Hospice   19

2. The Hospice Philosophy of Care   31

3. The Hospice Approach to Medical Treatment
   for the Person with AIDS   43

4. Emotional and Social Issues Related to
   Hospice Care for the Person with AIDS   59

5. How to Develop Hospice Programs
   for Persons with AIDS   75

7

8   Among Friends

6. Hospice Care for Children with AIDS
   (with Connie Wolf)   93

7. The Cost of Care for Persons with AIDS
   Mary Derby   115

8. Suicide, the Person with AIDS, and Hospice Care   139

Epilogue: A Chorus of Friends
   Ralph O. Hall   151

Glossary of Medical Terms   179

Select Bibliography   189

Acknowledgments

I wish to acknowledge three special people who helped make this book what it is. These people put much "sweat and tears" in their respective chapters. They are Mary Derby, Connie Wolf, and Ralph Hall. Each added his or her own special touch to make a contribution to the field of hospice care for the person with AIDS.

I also wish to acknowledge two magnificent women, Diane Fix and Karrie Riley. I labor and laugh with them every day. The road to any task's completion is covered with obstacles. Whenever I needed their support they were there for me; they have always made my job easier. These two women are interpersonal magicians who removed the obstacles so that I might proceed safely and successfully to my final destination. Without Diane and Karrie this book would not have been. I also would like to thank general services at Mankato State University for their aid in manuscript preparation.

And last but not least, I would like to thank Dan Wasinger, Steven Mitchell, and Eugene O'Connor of Prometheus Books. Without their vision and concern for the person with AIDS, this book would not be.

Prologue

Lessons from My Patient-Teachers

It is a cold, gray, bone-chilling morning in a midwestern winter. I am sitting looking at an early winter snow. Winter, especially here in Minnesota, is quite harsh: the trees are bare, and occasionally I see a deer traverse the snowy landscape. It is a time for reflection.

Reflection brings sadness as well as other things to consider. I ponder the fate of this book: Will it affect people? Will it be lost on the dusty shelf of some library or will it enlighten people as to the benefits of hospice care for the person with AIDS? I hope the latter. It is 1992. Ten years ago, many Americans were healing their emotional wounds from Vietnam. The memory, sadness, and the emotional pain of that war, in which 53,000 American lives had been lost, was coming to an end for most of us. The 1980s were to be a time for healing. But a tragedy far greater than the Vietnam War quietly and blindly struck the American people with awesome power: our first case of AIDS was diagnosed.

In the decade since, I report to you sadly that over 130,000 American lives have been lost to this epidemic.* It is estimated that

---

*As estimated by the Center for Disease Control in Atlanta, Georgia, as of November 1991.

one million Americans have been infected with the AIDS virus, most of whom do not know they carry it. When we think of the wars of the world, we think of great tragedies, great losses. There is no greater tragedy today than this horrible epidemic that is sweeping not only our country but the world. It is truly the "black plague" of the twentieth century. All that I can only offer now are words and advice for education, prevention, and the hope that soon we will have a vaccine and cure for this disease. This book revolves around my work with over 1,700 cancer and AIDS patients who have faced a terminal diagnosis. This work also focuses on my experiences in developing hospice programs for the person with AIDS throughout this country, the (former) Soviet Union, and Cuba. This book was written for caregivers, for people with AIDS, and for health professionals.

Recent news brought the tragic information that one of our leading NBA basketball stars and an American popular hero, Magic Johnson, has been infected with the AIDS virus, apparently through heterosexual contact. All at once, in one sweeping moment, the nation stood up and listened. A bolt of lightning struck the intellectual core of the American people. Could it be? Is this a disease that can affect and infect those of us who are heterosexual? We must face the fact that this is not just a disease specific to homosexuals, IV-drug users, or hemophiliacs, but one that threatens us all.

This is my seventh book. As a professor of medicine for fifteen years and now as a college dean of a state university in Minnesota, I write this book for those of you out there with an interest or concern for people with AIDS. Working with terminally ill cancer and AIDS patients for many years, I have obtained much wisdom from them, wisdom that I would like to share with you. The following "Lessons from Dr. Buckingham" are lessons from my patient-teachers.

Lesson No. 1: *Keep your life simple.* Many people have a tendency to complicate their lives with trivial matters and pursuits. It is very important to look at your life and not get wrapped up with insignificant trivia. Be able to focus on what really is important. What are your interests? What are your loves? Don't worry about things that you cannot change. Worry about the things that you can change.

Lesson No. 2: *Ask yourself three basic questions.* I have stated often to my medical and undergraduate students that there are *three basic questions* we must ask ourselves. They are: (1) Who am I? (2) What do I want? and (3) Where do I want to go? At different times in our lives we will have different answers to these questions, but the answers are not as important as remembering to ask the questions.

Lesson No. 3: *Eliminate the disadvantage complex.* The disadvantage complex is something that people say to themselves, subconsciously or consciously, like, "I'm too old," "I'm not smart enough," "I'm not attractive enough," or "I'm too fat." No one is too old, we are all of basically equal intelligence, and attraction is broad. We must not compare ourselves to others.

Lesson No. 4: *Challenge yourself.* It is important that we all try at times to challenge ourselves. For us to become stronger, to face another day, we must not become complacent with our being. Without self-challenge there is no growth. So many Americans are content to sit by their television set and to be entertained into a state of lethargy. There is so much going on outside our windows: so much to do, to see, and to feel. We must not be afraid of the challenge presented by new opportunities.

Lesson No. 5: *Do not compare yourself to others.* As I said earlier, it is very difficult to go on with our lives, to make them fruitful, if we are always comparing ourselves to others. It is a simple lesson: you are special. As you know, we can't compare oranges to apples; every human is different. Many of us are brought up with our parents always telling us things like, "Oh, I wish you could be as smart as little Johnny" or "I wish you could be as polite as little Suzy." It is a wrong lesson to learn. Take pride in your uniqueness. Do not be afraid to be who you are.

Lesson No. 6: *Maintain a positive outlook.* In life there are three kinds of people: those who say, "Things are going to be okay"; those who say, "Things are not going to be okay"; and those who say, "Whatever will be will be." We want to be the people for whom everything will be okay. Positive thoughts will become affirmations of our being; without them we cannot affirm the glory of our being or our becoming.

Lesson No. 7: *Stop complaining.* As a university professor for all these years, I have listened to students complaining every day: "This class is boring," "This professor is boring," "This professor doesn't care," "My boss doesn't care; he/she does not treat me nicely." If we listen to those around us, we will always hear people complaining. These are people, I think, who are focused on the minus signs of life, and who like to wallow in their own self-pity and negativism. They are slowly digging a hole for themselves. Don't fall into this trap. Stop your complaining. When you have problems—and we all do—it is important for us to look up and say, very simply, "It will pass, it will pass."

Lesson No. 8: *Be here now.* This is one great lesson I have learned from my patients who face the challenges of cancer and AIDS. It, too, is a simple lesson. Today is our most precious possession. Do not look back fondly to memories of yesterday or ahead to the possibilites of tomorrow; focus on the importance of becoming today, being today, being here now. Remember, life is only so long. No matter how long it is, it is never long enough. In one of my books I stated, "The greatest tragedy in life is not that we are going to die; the greatest tragedy in life is not living life fully." Now is the time to focus on. Be here now. Enjoy every moment you have.

Lesson No. 9: *You are responsible for your own happiness.* Do not expect others to bring it to you. Again, the ability to be content and happy lies within ourselves. It is a matter of self-responsibility, of internal signals and not external feedback.

Lesson No. 10: *Keep the craziness in you alive.* I like this lesson. Simply stated, don't lose touch with the craziness in you. All of us walk the fine line between normality and acceptance on the one hand, and, on the other, the little "crazy" thoughts we have. These thoughts might sometimes seem immature, silly, or insignificant. Sometimes they become actions. It's okay to be a little crazy, to laugh at yourself and the world. Keep this craziness alive in yourself. Wallow in it. It's fun. Remember, life is meant to be enjoyed. It's not serious business all the time.

Lesson No. 11: *Let go of your anger, hurt, or pain.* I have learned this lesson with my patients' families. Do not hold on to anger, hurt, or pain. They will only take away your energy for loving life. Don't let your anger and pain stay inside you very long. Deal with them, speak about them, but don't be afraid to let them go.

Lesson No. 12: *Adventure through your life.* This is probably the most important lesson. It is vital that we look at life as an adventure, no matter how long we have. There are so many wonderful things that we can do, so many wonderful people we can touch and love. The greatest adventure in life is loving and enjoying other people.

I would like to go on now with a few more lessons I have learned from my patient-teachers. They have taught me to understand what love is. Quite simply, they have taught me that to love successfully you must live your life the way you choose. By that I mean you must be able to stand up for your beliefs; you must not be monitored by the dictates and beliefs of others. Many of us handicap ourselves by a lack of self-confidence. But we must draw strength from ourselves and not let other people victimize us. You see so many people in America today who seem content just being regulated by others. They don't want to take charge of their own lives.

You must say, "This is my life. I choose to be happy. I choose to be depressed. I choose to be sad. I choose to be positive. I choose to be in love. I choose to be without love. I choose to be strong. I choose to succeed. I choose to be weak. I choose to fail." We might victimize ourselves because we've convinced ourselves that some people won't like us or that disaster is around the corner. Be careful of these thoughts. They can take away your effectiveness and future success. Thoughts like this will betray your internal support system. The bravest thing you can do when you have thoughts like these is to profess courage and act accordingly. In what I call the professing of courage I am referring to statements like, "I can do it," "I will be liked," "I will be accepted," "I am strong." You must remove and eliminate the disadvantage complex.

Another word of advice—stay away from people who want you to join them in their misery. So many depressed and sad souls are only looking for others to whom they can tell their story or on whom they can unload their baggage. Remember, these people can zap your courage.

Another lesson I have learned from people who have a dread disease and a short time to live is that we should not victimize others. By this I am referring to making such statements as, "I don't understand why you say those things," "How could you do such a thing," "How could anyone with your brains and background do such a thing," "Do it for me," "You've offended me," "I demand an apology." Avoid making such victimizing statements. They will not help your relationships with others. And never place loyalty to institutions and things above loyalty to yourself. Remember, as Shakespeare said, "This above all, to thine own self be true, for it shall follow as the night the day: thou shan't be false to any man."

Remember that life is a continuous series of experiences rather than one single experience. I believe that our successes can only be measured by our constant motivation, perseverance, and a number of failures. I believe we must fail to succeed. Remember, for us to live fully we must learn to use things and to love people, not love things and use people.

In closing I would like to make a very simple comment about life itself. Humankind, unlike the other animals, has either forgotten or has never learned that the sole purpose of life is to enjoy it. We must reach out, touch it, enjoy it, live it, and love it. Again, we must look at the opportunities that we have today. Make today count and don't ever forget to count your blessings.

DR. BUCKINGHAM'S ADVICE TO THE CAREGIVER

1. Expect to invest a great deal of time and energy in your patient relationship.

2. Remember that a patient-caregiver relationship is a pooling of resources. That means that with each relationship you are not only giving, you are becoming more.

3. Don't think in terms of forever. Think of now, and forever will take care of itself.

4. Remove the price tag from your patients. Everyone has worth. The excitement lies in determining their value.

5. Don't allow the experience of death to load down your heart. Use it to become more aware and sensitive.

6. See all people as good and beautiful until proven otherwise.

7. Value yourself.

8. Learn to bend. It is better than breaking.

9. Don't take yourself too seriously. Share laughter and humor with your patients.

10. Expect what is reasonable from your patients, not what is perfect.

11. Don't hold on to your anger or pain. It steals your energy for doing good.

12. Don't lose touch with the child in you. Mixing humor with compassion will assure that you will never become boring to your patients.

13. Keep the child in you alive.

14. Don't allow anyone to put you on a pedestal. It is too easy to fall off.

Robert W. Buckingham
Good Thunder, Minnesota
January 1992

1

The History of Hospice

"Hospitality," "hospitable," "host," "hostess," "hospital," "hostel," "hotel," "hospice"—all these words have the same root, the Latin word *hospes.* All include the ideas of kindness and generosity to strangers, or caring for our fellow beings and offering them nourishment and refreshment.

Ancient hospices or hospitals (the two were one for a number of centuries) provided sanctuary for the poor wayfarer, the sick and dying, the woman in labor, the orphan, the needy, and the religious pilgrim. Medieval hospices were generally run by religious orders, serving the Lord by serving His poor, His sick, and those in need of shelter. Welcome was extended to wayfarers by hospices throughout Europe in major towns and cities, in villages, in remote monastic hermitages, and along the route to the Holy Land. The Knights Hospitallers of the Order of St. John of Jerusalem in the twelfth century A.D. offered aid to pilgrims and the sick throughout Europe, and at one time were active and held land in Rhodes, Cyprus, Italy, Germany, and England. If hospice workers were unkind to patients, or neglected them in any way, the workers were whipped and condemned to eat bread and water for a week.[1] The records of the

19

Knights Hospitallers, kept for six hundred years, show their efforts to maintain their ideals and goals, despite increasing wealth and land holdings. At their hospice, or hospital, in Rhodes, the incurably ill were sheltered and cared for in a group of rooms reserved for travelers and pilgrims, apart from those with other illnesses.

Since, in the medieval worldview, life and death were each considered part of the same mortal process, pilgrims and travelers were housed together with the dying. All were on a journey, and therefore needed a place to stop for comfort. The news the travelers brought with them from the outside world was of value; the dying were also valued as individuals and as beings who were on the road to a higher plane of existence.

With the forced closure of monasteries in many countries during the Reformation, the concepts of hospice and hospital gradually became distinct. Today, the responsibility of caring for the sick and dying, formerly a private or religious one, has become a public, or government, function.[2] Although science has supported medicine with marvelous discoveries to cure disease and prolong life, the modern hospital increasingly has the look and feel of a laboratory. The bureaucracy needed to support the hospital system places increasing demands on the time and energy of medical staff as well as patients. The modern hospital, though well equipped to aid in an acute, life-threatening situation, is seldom in a position to offer comfort to a traveler who is nearing his or her journey's end. Now, after a lapse of several centuries, hospices are again caring for the dying and their families, due in large part to the work of Cicely Saunders in England and Elisabeth Kübler-Ross in the United States.

In the late 1940s, Dr. Saunders became friends with a man in his forties, who was dying of cancer in a busy London hospital. As they talked, the idea of a place that could meet the needs of the dying—his needs—began to grow. Together they shared the dream of a haven where others like him could die in peace and dignity. This man, who had escaped from the Warsaw ghetto, died in 1948; he bequeathed £500 to Dr. Saunders in order to be, as he put it, "a window in your Home."[3]

St. Christopher's Hospice* grew from this gift, and from the work and planning of other donors over the next decade. St. Christopher's has continued to expand its services, including a Domiciliary Service Program, which educates staff, students, and visitors; it is from this model that other hospices have grown, both in England and in the United States. Financial needs are met partly by contracts with the National Health Service, with the remainder being made up by donations. True to the old hospice ideal, no patient is refused service because of inability to pay. "Giving care is St. Christopher's only way of fund raising."[4]

Patients with various terminal illnesses are admitted to the hospice at their doctors' request. Some come to stay, while others remain for a time, then return home; a few who have shown an improvement are sent back to a treatment hospital. Whatever the disease or the prognosis, all patients receive personal care and are greeted by name upon admission and throughout their stay. Bereaved families are supported by visits from St. Christopher's staff and volunteers. Relatives of deceased patients are remembered with anniversary cards the first year after bereavement, and are welcome to services at the chapel and to a monthly social club, as well as to general parties attended by staff and their families. Like residents of a small village, St. Christopher's staff, patients, and families share a feeling of community, a family feeling.

Dr. Saunders visited Yale University in the early 1960s to speak of her efforts on behalf of the terminally ill. With St. Christopher's now in full operation, a group of clergymen and medical people in New Haven, Connecticut, began making efforts to develop an American hospice. Florence Wald, R.N., former dean of the Yale University School of Nursing, investigated the need for hospice in New Haven. Reverend Edward Dobihal, clinical professor of pastoral care at Yale Divinity School and director of religious ministries at the Yale-New Haven Hospital, who had long been concerned about the care of the terminally ill in his ministry, also contributed to the study, which was finished in late 1969. The next few years saw incor-

---

*The name "hospice" had been revived by the Irish Sisters of Charity, who began opening homes for dying patients in the nineteenth century.

poration, the formulation of a hospice philosophy, and a donation enabling Hospice of New Haven to rent a small office and to hire Florence Wald and three others. Later, Dr. Syliva Lack of St. Christopher's was hired as the first medical director.

Progress was slow, however. When local opposition prohibited land purchase for a facility, the founders realized they needed to prepare and educate the public to receive hospice. Approval came gradually. By mid-1974, patients were being served by the home-care program, and in autumn of the same year, funds were received from the National Cancer Institute and the Kaiser Foundation.* By late 1976, the community had given its full support.

The New Haven hospice was the first of three demonstration projects funded by the National Cancer Institute; the others were located in Boonton, New Jersey, and Tucson, Arizona. Two fundamental difficulties had to be faced: the American medical community's existing terminal care policy and the bureaucracy of contemporary health care. Planners feared that hospice ideals and goals would be compromised. Indeed, many in the medical establishment expressed doubts at first, thinking that hospice, and palliative home care particularly, would be unacceptable in this country. Planners were told that "when Americans are sick, they want to be in a hospital. Nobody dies at home in this country; the society isn't set up for it."[5]

But the response of patients and families has proved otherwise. A service emphasizing care rather than technology can be accepted by both laypeople and professionals. Evaluation studies done at the time (1974–1976, when I was director of research at a hospice) show that hospice services measurably benefit patients and families. In a quasi-experimental control study I conducted as a dissertation for the Yale School of Medicine, I found that primary-care persons who had had hospice support showed less anxiety and hostility than those who had not. Hospice, Inc., New Haven, and the National Cancer Institute have demonstrated that many people in this country do desire home care and are willing to make sacrifices and adjustments in order to keep a family member at home.

---

*A health maintenance organization in California

Since Hospice Inc., New Haven, began serving patients in 1974, the concept has spread rapidly. Communities throughout the country have sought hospice services and are creating facilities. The National Hospice Organization's (NHO) 1990 directory lists 138 member organizations providing service, with present estimates running as high as 800 for hospices in varying stages of development.

Hospice is a flexible concept that can fit into many settings. Some hospices are functioning today with a base in an established hospital; others have independent inpatient facilities, or affiliations with another community service. Not all American hospices offer inpatient care, but home care and bereavement programs seem to be the norm. It appears that two divergent types of hospices are developing: (1) independent, heavily volunteer hospices with unstable funding, in which a variety of professional staff deliver a wide array of social and psychological services; and (2) institutionally based hospices providing both inpatient and home care, supplying a greater variety of medical/nursing services but fewer social/psychological services; the latter employ a smaller number of volunteers and paid staff, and experience no funding problems. A recent study that I undertook with Dale Lupu[6] indicates that the funding mix varies considerably from program to program. Private sources (individuals and foundations) provide support to a majority of hospices; third-party contributors (private carriers, Medicare, Medicaid, and state and local government) also help, despite the lack of any specific national public programs to reimburse such services as physician home visits, pastoral care, volunteer directors, homemakers, and education.

Even in the face of funding difficulties, the hospice concept is well and thriving in the 1990s. Congress recently voted to extend Medicare coverage to hospice care (mainly because it is less expensive than hospitals or nursing homes). Though such coverage is limited, it indicates national recognition of the widely held value of the hospice concept. In less than a decade since the first hospice patients began to be cared for in New Haven, the concept had achieved such recognition that President Ronald Reagan declared November 7–14, 1982, National Hospice Week in order to encourage government agencies, the medical community, private organizations, and citizens to participate in a "national recognition and support for the hospice care concept." The hospice idea is springing up and taking root in our time, as in ages past. Hospices are already flourishing in Canada, Japan, Italy, Denmark, and Sweden.

WHY DO WE NEED HOSPICE?

Although it is a cliché to say that today we live in a highly techno-logical, bureaucratic society in which community and personal supports and traditions have broken down, nonetheless it's true. The needs of the dying and their families are personal, and those needs are not often met by the impersonal, highly specialized medical technology and the bureaucracy of the modern acute care hospital.

Care should enable the terminally ill to continue as vital functioning participants in life, and to maintain their identity and capacity to contribute as full human beings. Unfortunately, dying patients are often cared for in acute care hospitals and institutional settings, where the structure, organization, and philosophy of the medical staff are geared toward aggressive cure. Practices in such facilities characteristically exclude the elements that are essential in the delivery of proper terminal care: involvement of the family in the patient's medical situation, which facilitates acceptance and alleviates potential guilt; care of the patient and family with respect to all relevant needs—physical, emotional, spiritual, and social; avoidance of heroic measures when such treatments are not warranted by the prognosis; effective use of narcotics for the alleviation of pain; execution of the patient's wishes with respect to environment and therapy options; and integration of the medical staff as a unified team into the process of maintaining the patient's total well-being.

There is general accord among those examining current practices in the care of the terminally ill that existing institutional practice is usually deficient, inappropriate, limited, and in many cases devastating to the patient. David Shephard cites three reasons for the pervasive inadequacy of terminal care.[7] First, the emphasis on treatment and investigation leads the medical staff to regard the patient as a disease entity and not as a whole person. As Kübler-Ross has indicated, the patient "may cry for rest, peace, and dignity but he will get infusions, transfusions, a heart machine or tracheotomy, if necessary."[8] The patients are often inappropriately subjected to the rigors of curative therapy even when they are beyond the stage of possible recovery; at this time, whatever therapy is given should instead be geared solely to maximizing comfort. A second factor in deficient terminal care is treatment in an inappropriate environment. In an acute care hospital, the orientation of facilities, policies, and staff is toward cure rather than alleviating suffering, whereas a hospice is by nature dedicated to meeting the everyday needs of its patients. Inadequate care may also be a consequence of the psychological inability of people in our society to confront the dying. Ironically, investigators have found that physicians are more fearful of death than members of any other occupation. Herman Feifel suggests that practicing curative medicine facilitates and reinforces the denial of death, thereby preventing physicians from comforting their patients and providing nonclinical, social, and personal support.[9]

The third factor underlying inadequate care in a health-care environment is the training of the staff, which exacerbates rather than alleviates society's inability to confront or cope with death. Dehumanizing approaches to patient care result when staff anxieties intervene in the process of assisting the dying person. Defensive behavior by staff and friends, such as indifference, hostility, or detachment from the dying person, magnifies the loneliness of hospitalization and accentuates the withdrawal of the patient, who is already experiencing a diminished sense of self and a decreasing awareness of the environment. Interaction between patient and staff are strained further by the pressure of bureaucratic hospital procedures.

The tendency to quietly forget about patients once they are stigmatized with the label "incurable" can bring on a terrible sense of desolation. Patients may become overwhelmed with hopelessness, withdrawing into loneliness and depression.

Death in the acute care setting represents a technological failure, not a natural and inevitable conclusion to life. Fortunately, due in part to the positive effects of Elisabeth Kübler-Ross's work, attitudes toward death are being reexamined, and with new attitudes may come a more humane and sensible approach to the care of the dying. To accomplish this completely, changes must be made in medical education. Unfortunately, although many enter medical professions for humanitarian reasons, doctors are often trained to cure, not to care. "What's happening in our medical schools and hospitals these days?" asks Dr. Morris Wessel, clinical professor of pediatrics at Yale University School of Medicine and a founding member of the New Haven Hospice. "You walk to the door, you leave your humanity outside. . . . Why did physicians stop paying attention to the human side of the patient? . . . We need to stop separating our professional functions into little niches in the hospital and in the medical schools, in the office or home. . . . The young doctors today need to understand that human beings die. It happens; that's reality."[10] Caring is healing, no matter how long the patient lives.

Hospices have an educational effect upon physicians. When the hospice is not housed in a hospital, there is a great opportunity to learn about palliative care, about the value of home visits and of interacting with dying patients. Physicians who continue to care for their patients after referral to an independent hospice are also learning these techniques. Naturally, other aspects of their practice are affected as well. With the comfort *and* cure of the patient in mind, physicians and nurses become willing to learn about symptom control from hospice.

As the comfort of the patient is one of the prime reasons for the existence of hospice, it is also one of the reasons for hospice's popularity. Besides, many people prefer to die at home rather that in an institution. The patient's comfort does not rely exclusively on medications for pain, or on corrective measures for distressing symptoms; it is also drawn from the environment—being comfortable, having familiar surroundings, loving care, and perhaps two kinds of visitors seldom seen in an acute care setting: young children and pets. Comfort may also mean the freedom to live and die in the style of life that the patient has created.

The comfort of familiar surroundings, or a homelike inpatient hospice unit, benefits the family also. The patient in distress is not the only one suffering; the family suffers as well. One of the basic tenets of hospice care is the treatment of patient and family together. Death in acute care institutions has caused many families to come apart; hospice helps to make death a coming together. Approaching death can be spiritual and growth-filled, an experience families can share. Hospice staff are trained to facilitate communication between family members so that the remaining time can be as complete as possible. Family problems cannot be ignored, for if they remain unresolved, they affect the peace of the dying person. When family members are able to express feelings, patients feel less isolated and freer to express their feelings.

Caring for the patient at home decreases any feelings of guilt the family may have. Even when a patient is cared for in an inpatient hospice unit, the staff encourages family members to attend the patient. Again, training one or more family members as primary care persons lessens the anxiety and stress of patient and family. The family members know that they have done everything they were capable of doing for the patient's comfort.

Caring for the patient at home also affords survivors protection from the hazards of bereavement. A recent study indicates that a significant difference exists in the mortality experience of grieving families, depending upon whether the patient died at home or in the hospital. The risk of the remaining relative dying within a year of bereavement was found to double if the first death occurred in a hospital rather than at home.[11] For those cases in which the patient has been cared for at home prior to death, the ability of family members to resist a devastating and prolonged period of grief is attributable to the continuing support of professionals who assisted in the care of the patient, to lessened difficulty in accepting the reality of the loved one's death by those who witnessed the progression of the illness, and to the value of anticipatory grief.

The terminally ill person who is dying at home is still part of the community, a community of neighbors of varying ages and occupations, from the postman to a visiting toddler. It is beneficial for relatives and children to witness the dying process at home, and not be frightened of it. A positive experience at home can counteract the unnatural scenes of violent death that saturate the media. Many who have been present during a peaceful death fear their own mortality less.

After death has occurred, surviving family members receive continued care from hospice. Hospices in the United States and in England offer individual bereavement support, follow-up visits by hospice staff, and bereavement groups. This helps to prevent some of the loneliness that exacerbates grief. Mourners often experience isolation, and do not receive much understanding or tolerance from the rest of society. After the first flurry of activity following a death, the bereaved are likely to be left alone, and are expected to return to "normal" within a short time. We are beginning to recognize, however, along with changing attitudes toward death, that mourning is a necessary psychological process which can be aided by acknowledgment from the rest of the community. Hospices are invaluable in this process, for the family, as the unit of care, is not abandoned after a member's death. The bereavement process cannot be avoided or curtailed, but it can be resolved by continuity of care.

We often think of the dying as "them" and the living as "us," as if we were separate. Among the moral and spiritual benefits of caring for a dying family member is the erasure of this distinction. We are all on the same journey, come from the same entrance, and leave by the same exit. We are all wayfarers on the road, and all of us need to stop for refreshment and comfort before the end of our journey. With hospice, we now have a choice about where and how we would like that stop to be.

NOTES

1. Sandol Stoddard, *The Hospice Movement* (New York: Stein and Day, 1978), p. 91.

2. Ibid., p. 40.

3. Herman Feifel, *New Meanings of Death* (New York: McGraw-Hill, 1977), p. 159.

4. Ibid., p. 161

5. Sylvia Lack and Robert W. Buckingham, *First American Hospice: Three Years of Home Care* (New Haven, Conn.: 1978), p. 4

6. Robert W. Buckingham and Dale Lupu, "A Comparative Study of Hospice Services in the United States," *American Journal of Public Health* 72 (May 1982): 455.

7. David Shephard, "Terminal Care: Towards an Ideal," *Canadian Medical Association Journal* 115 (July 1976): 97–98.

8. Elisabeth Kübler-Ross, *On Death and Dying* (New York: Macmillan, 1969), p. 9.

9. Herman Feifel, "Perception of Death," *Annals of the New York Academy of Science* 164 (1969): 669.

10. Stoddard, *The Hospice Movement,* pp. 141–42.

11. Dewi W. Rees and Sylvia G. Lutkins, "Mortality of Bereavement," *British Medical Journal* (October 1967).

2

The Hospice Philosophy of Care

Since the first American hospice home-care program was established in New Haven in 1974, hospice programs have been organized all over the country, with still more in development. Many types of people support hospice concepts, and now because of AIDS (Acquired Immunodeficiency Syndrome) and the large numbers of people affected, more people are taking a closer look at hospice programs.

Although there may be a significant time interval between initial infection (testing HIV positive) and actually contracting AIDS, and although strides have been made in prolonging the lives of persons with AIDS, the inescapable truth is that AIDS is a relentless disease and inevitably fatal. During December 1990, 3,496 confirmed cases, with 2,265 deaths, among adults and adolescents; and 52 cases, with 18 deaths, among children were reported to the U.S. Centers for Disease Control. Between the disease's initial outbreak in 1981 and December 1990, the number of people who have died of AIDS has reached 99,372. According to the January 1991 HIV/AIDS Surveillance Report from the Centers for Disease Control (1990), 158,287 cases of AIDS were reported among adults and adolescents in the United States through December 1990. For children younger than

31

thirteen, 2,786 cases have been reported. The majority of people with AIDS are young men and women in the third and fourth decades of their lives, who must resign themselves to the fact that, with no known cure or vaccine, they will die of this illness at a very early age.

An increasing number of people are seeking to use the hospice approach in the care of the terminally ill AIDS patient. This chapter will describe hospice, palliative care and curative care, the goals of hospice, and the hospice team. It will also discuss some of the barriers to hospice care.

DEFINITION

Hospice is primarily a philosophy of care and a program for the terminally ill. It is not necessarily a facility. The program can be carried out in the person's home, in a separate free-standing facility, in a department of a general acute care hospital, or as a separate facility attached either physically or organizationally to a general hospital.[1] The hospice approach centers on helping the dying and their loved ones to maintain the dignity and humaneness of the dying process and providing sophisticated medical and nursing care. The focus of the hospice approach and philosophy is to help the dying to live as fully as possible during the time that remains. Through the control of symptoms, hospice care seeks to eliminate the suffering that accompanies the dying process.[2]

Hospice care, however, goes beyond the elimination of symptoms. The focus is not on the disease itself, but on the patient and family. The hospice community makes every effort to provide appropriate care and to promote a caring community which is sensitive to the needs of the patients and families. It is hoped this will help them attain a degree of mental and spiritual preparedness for death.[3]

PALLIATIVE CARE VERSUS CURATIVE CARE

The health system is oriented toward the cure of disease. Physicians are taught to diagnose and treat disease with the expectation of cure as a consequence. This orientation ignores the fuller definition of medical care, which dates back to the fifteenth century—to cure sometimes, to relieve often, and to comfort always.[4] The cure of disease is not the goal of all medical therapy. Seen from a broader and more complete perspective, the goal of medical therapy is the provision of suitable treatment to the patient. Treatment is appropriate if the physician applies one of two complementary systems at the correct time: one concerned with eliminating a controllable disease and the other concerned with relieving the symptoms of an incurable illness. When cure is not possible, improving the quality of life of the patient through palliative care is the appropriate approach.[5] It is important to stress that palliative care does not simply mean the mitigation of suffering by symptom relief alone; it includes everything that hospice does to help the patient continue life in as near to a usual manner as possible. This means helping the patient and family to make the best use of the time they have left to share.[6]

THE GOALS OF HOSPICE

In a general hospital, the staff works toward the attainment of four basic goals: investigation, diagnosis, cure, and the prolongation of life. However, the goals of hospice are quite different. Hospices seek to provide relief from the distressing symptoms of the disease, the security of a caring environment, sustained expert care, and the assurance that patients and their families will not be abandoned.[7]

Symptom control is a major ingredient of hospice care. After physicians and nurses are able to determine the cause of the symptoms, attempts are made to apply treatment that will alleviate them and avoid unnecessary side effects. Because the competent hospice team is aware that the terminally ill patient has extremely low physical, physiological, and emotional reserves, the entire team—which includes the patient and family—chooses a treatment option that will not complicate patient management. Every effort will be made to prevent symptoms by applying appropriate therapies at intervals that maintain a continuing beneficial effect. Finally, symptom control demands continuous monitoring of the patient; this allows for immediate and proper changes in care by responding to changes in the patient's condition.[8]

A caring environment is essential to the hospice approach. The patient's entire spectrum of needs (physical, intellectual, emotional, social, financial, and spiritual) are addressed. Causes of happiness and distress for the patient and family are of concern to the hospice team.[9]

Hospice provides sustained expert care available around the clock, whenever the patient might require assistance, regardless of location.[10] Families are able to keep their relative at home due to the twenty-four-hour service availability offered by hospices. Care is provided by an expert team which includes the physician, nurse, social worker, family, and trained volunteers.

Finally, hospice provides the patient and the family with the assurance that they will not be abandoned. The feeling of abandonment is one of the major problems of terminally ill patients. Emotional support is an essential aspect of hospice care.[11] The emphasis is on making the process of dying a *coming-together* experience for the patient and family. Even after death has occurred, emotional support for the surviving family members continues. This may include individual bereavement support, follow-up visits by hospice staff, and bereavement groups.

THE HOSPICE TEAM

Care is provided for the terminally ill patient by a multidisciplinary patient care team comprised of everyone who participates in the patient's care: physician, nurses, social worker, physical therapist, pharmacologist, chaplain, volunteers, patient, and family. Because hospice care is personal, the team is shaped by the personal needs and preferences of each patient and family. The team meets together at least weekly to review each patient's and family's progress. Through these meetings they have the opportunity to share their perspectives regarding both assessment and management. This kind of team work enables each member to approach the patient and the family with a personal, hands-on understanding as well as a professional understanding of the contributions of all aspects of care. This cooperative approach allows hospice to provide its patients and families with a comprehensive program of care, and at the same time enables the team members to cope with the stress that is intrinsic to working with the grief and suffering of others.[12] Each team member plays an important and active role in caring for the patient. The roles of the physician, nurse, and volunteers will be described in more detail.

Physicians play a pivotal and crucial role in the program. First of all, they have a responsibility and authority, both professional and legal, which no other hospice team member has. The physician orders diagnostic studies and establishes a valid diagnosis, and is the only member of the team who has a license to prescribe medications that provide the most effective palliative care. Doctors also certify legal death and secure reimbursement for ancillary health care services. The team looks to the physician for assurance that it has satisfied its responsibilities in a medically competent and effective manner; the doctor guides program administration so that the hospice meets the needs of the patient and the family.[13,14]

In most home health agency or hospice programs, it is the *nurse* who assesses the patient's physical condition, provides interventions, and discusses with the physician relevant changes in the patient. Other responsibilities include teaching team members about infection control, pain and symptom management, and comfort measures. Because the course of AIDS is so unpredictable, the nurse must be on call twenty-four hours per day.[15]

What the nurse offers depends largely on the condition of the patient, the particular symptoms present in the illness, and the existing degree of independence. This care involves not only symptom and pain control, but also such items as bathing, control of odor, mouth care, care of hair, and bladder care. Depending on the setting, the nurse may take direct charge of some of these services, or they may be provided by attendants or volunteers. The nurse has the responsibility of caring for and closely observing the patient. Patients have to be taught to say when they are in pain or discomfort. The nurse must be able to anticipate pain and thus keep the patient as pain-free as possible.[16] Hospice nurses, working within physicians' prescriptions for dose ranges and flexible intervals, have effectively and safely adjusted the dosages of pain medications for patients who have prolonged, variable, and sometimes severe pain.[17]

Volunteers play a large role in bringing about the high level of personal care found in hospices. They are carefully interviewed, trained, and screened before placement on a hospice team. Listening and communication skills are primary, along with an understanding of the humane philosophies that are fundamental to the program.

Volunteers may serve in a variety of positions: direct care givers, receptionists, public speakers, photographers and writers, and researchers. A good volunteer gets to know the patient and family and becomes a friend, which may be one of the most important functions of a volunteer. The patient and family often need the support and relief that the volunteer can offer. Many times it is easier for the patient and family to relate to and to confide in a volunteer than it is for them to deal with a professional. Also, when a relationship develops during an illness, the volunteer may become an important visitor during bereavement.

Volunteers bring fresh outlooks to hospice and provide energy and support that the program needs in order to exist. Although volunteers do not replace paid staff, they do supplement hospice services and provide needed support to the patient, the family, and to other team members. Volunteers are important people in hospice care and largely contribute to making hospice a caring community.

By participating in a hospice program, each team member will have the opportunity to learn from the other members, each of whom brings special perspectives to the program. For a hospice program to be effective, there must be intense internal communication, both professionally and personally, among all team members.

ADVANTAGES OF HOSPICE CARE
OVER CONVENTIONAL CARE

Although the philosophy of hospice care is appealing, studies addressing its advantages over those of conventional care have yielded mixed results. The National Hospice Study followed up 1,754 terminal cancer patients in 40 hospices (20 hospital-based and 20 home care) and 14 conventional care settings from 1981 through 1983. The study found that the quality of life was similar for patients in hospice and conventional care. Inpatient hospices provided somewhat better pain and symptom control than conventional care or home care hospices. Hospice care patients were more likely to die at home. Although family members appreciated the fact that the patient was able to remain at home, they were under more stress in home care hospices. A secondary analysis of the study found that the quality of death (the last three days of life) was significantly better for hospice patients than for patients who received conventional care. The items focused upon were those that the patients saw as important, such as freedom from pain and the ability to stay home as long as possible.[18]

At a Department of Veterans Affairs hospital, a study of terminal cancer patients randomly assigned to receive either hospice care or conventional care found no significant differences in pain control, symptom control, or functional ability. Yet, hospice patients expressed more satisfaction with their care and had greater involvement in that care than conventional care patients. Also, a study of twelve hospices in New York State found high overall levels of satisfaction with the provision of services and emotional support to the primary care provider, the effect on the patient's physical and emotional well-being, the home care services provided, and bereavement services. Although the satisfaction with community-based programs was high, it was lower than that for hospital-based programs.[19]

A conclusion to be drawn from the studies to date is that patient and caregiver satisfaction with hospice care is at least comparable to and often superior to that with conventional care. However, the reduction of patient pain and caregiver stress appears to be more effective in inpatient units than in home care-based programs.[20] Family caregivers are able to leave inpatient facilities for home and thus have time away from a stressful situation; this might not be possible in a home care situation.

Case Study

"Michael," a forty-three-year-old black gay man with a two-month diagnosis of AIDS, was admitted to the AIDS Home Care and Hospice program following discharge from the hospital. He had received treatment for PCP (Pneumocystis carinii pneumonia), esophageal candidiasis, and multiple other ailments. The nurse and social worker made their first visit together. The nurse made an assessment of Michael's physical complaints by reviewing his medical history and performing a physical examination. Michael, who had been a large-framed man weighing over 200 pounds, now weighed a mere 120 pounds and suffered from severe wasting of his skeletal muscles combined with sensory changes. He could barely stand.

Michael agreed to the nurse visiting daily for dressing changes and physical assessment. The social worker visited every two weeks for assistance with community resources. Michael also had an attendant for personal care and light housekeeping. A physical therapist helped him with the chore of moving around his apartment.

After Michael's condition continued to decline, the team was able to maintain him at home through additional services and financial support. When his dehydration worsened with persistent diarrhea and anorexia, the physician ordered intravenous fluids administered at home. Michael's breathing became even more labored; it was treated with oral morphine and oxygen. While Michael received medical care, the social worker followed up with in-depth counseling. He arranged for Michael's mother to fly out for a visit. While she was there, Michael said prayers with her. A pastor from the local church made a home visit for spiritual support. Michael died peacefully with a nurse and two hospice volunteers present. Hospice allowed Michael to have choice in his life and in his dying. Despite suffering from all the ravages of AIDS, he maintained his dignity at home and was surrounded by the people he trusted.[21]

BARRIERS TO HOSPICE CARE

Hospices now serve only a small peercentage of terminally ill patients. Medicare hospice benefits are used by far fewer people than originally projected—less than 13,000 in 1985, compared with a projected number of 40,000. There are several reasons for this underutilization. First, a relatively small number of hospices have sought Medicare certification. There are five main reasons that qualified hospices do not seek such certification:

(1) Medicare requires that the physician certify that the patient will die within six months. The course of advanced malignancy is considered easier to predict than that of other serious illnesses, but errors in prognosis are common, usually on the side of overestimating life expectancy. Predicting the course of diseases other than cancers may be even more inaccurate, making appropriate referral difficult. AIDS, which was first considered to be an invariably fatal and rapidly progressive disease, is now becoming a chronic progressive illness. Death is caused by an intercurrent infection,* and the patient may survive if the infection is treated aggressively. This may help explain why many patients are referred to hospice in the final days or even hours of life, when hospice care is unlikely to be of much benefit to the patient or the family. The most common reason for not admitting patients referred to hospices is death before care can be arranged.

(2) Medicare requires that hospices directly provide medical, nursing, social work, and counseling services and obtain contracts with hospitals for inpatient services.

(3) Medicare places aggregate payment caps and limits on inpatient stays.

(4) Payment is limited to 210 days.

(5) Pay rates are inadequate.[22]

---

*That is, an infection contracted by a patient who already has an infection or other diseases.

Another reason for the underutilization of hospices is that Medicare and individual hospices place limits on the patients who are admitted. Many Medicare-certified hospices require each patient to have a twenty-four-hour caregiver. This limits hospice care for those who are lacking in strong family supports and financial resources, but it is these patients who are most in need of hospice. In the National Hospice Study, patients who selected hospital-based hospices were more likely to live alone, to have less support at home, and to be more functionally dependent than those entering home care hospices. Home hospice patients tend to be younger and to have stronger family supports compared with other dying patients. Medicare-certified hospices will also tend to exclude patients who require expensive care and/or medications. AIDS patients who are receiving the drug AZT* might be denied admission because the hospice is concerned about the cost.

A third reason for the underutilization of hospice programs is that many people are unaware of the available services.

Finally, medical and nursing education is another barrier to effective use of the hospice in the community. Many doctors and nurses have not been trained to care for the terminally ill. In addition, medical professionals are not comfortable with the role of caring for the dying. Because of the lack of education in pain control in most medical training, fear of addiction is common.[23]

CONCLUSION

With an understanding of the hospice philosophy, it is easy to see why an increasing number of people are opting for such programs. The care and sense of community created by the hospice team may be very beneficial to the persons with AIDS and concerned family members. It is important for terminal patients to live the rest of their lives to the fullest, to maintain their identity, and to have the capacity to contribute as full human beings.

AIDS is the final stage of infection with HIV and on the average

*zidovudine

it takes ten years to develop. Because of this time period, many AIDS cases will arise in the years to come from all of the HIV-infected persons. Although future efforts may be successful in slowing the spread of HIV, many people have already been infected with the virus. The World Health Organization projects that by the year 2000, there will be 40 million HIV infections worldwide.[24]

With this knowledge, it is essential for health-care professionals, families, and communities to understand the dying process and to be able to approach it in a healthy light. Many of us will be faced with the reality that a family member, friend, or neighbor is dying of AIDS. When we are with our loved ones as they reach the end of their lives, we feel not only a loss for ourselves but also a sadness for them. Life, at least as we know it, is ebbing away for them. We can only hope for competent and caring professionals who can enable the dying to leave this world with dignity and who can lend support to those of us left behind. The hospice philosophy is an answer to that hope.

NOTES

1. K. P. Cohen, *Hospice, Prescription of Terminal Care* (Germantown, Md.: Aspen Systems Corporation, 1979), pp. 2–3.

2. D. C. McKell, "Hospice Care—A New Concept for the Care of the Terminally Ill and Their Families," workshop at UCLA Extension, Los Angeles, April, 1978.

3. C. A. Corr and D. M. Corr, *Hospice Care: Principles and Practice* (New York: Springer Publishing Co., 1983), p. 105.

4. Ibid., p. 104.

5. D. A. E. Shephard, "Principles and Practice of Palliative Care," *Canadian Medical Association Journal* 116 (1977): 522–26.

6. Ibid., p. 106.

7. Cohen, *Hospice, Prescription of Terminal Care,* pp. 3–4.

8. Corr and Corr, *Hospice Care: Principles and Practice,* p. 109.

9. Ibid., p. 108.

10. Ibid.

11. Ibid., p. 109.

12. Ibid., p. 110.

13. Ibid., pp. 111–16.

14. W. Bulkin and H. Lukashok, "Rx for Dying: The Case for Hospice," *The New England Journal of Medicine* 318 (1988): 377–78.

15. J. P. Martin, "Hospice and Home Care for Persons with AIDS/ARC," *Death Studies* 12 (1988): 468–69.

16. Corr and Corr, *Hospice Care: Principles and Practice,* pp. 123–27.

17. M. McCaffery, "Pain Management: Nurses Lead the Way to New Priorities," *American Journal of Nursing* 90 (1990): 45-46.

18. J. Rhymes, "Hospice Care in America," *Journal of the American Medical Association* 264 (1990): 370.

19. Ibid.

20. Ibid.

21. C. Clark, A. Curley, A. Hughes, and R. James, "Hospice Care: A Model for Caring for the Person with AIDS," *Nursing Clinics of North America* 23 (1988): 859–60.

22. Rhymes, "Hospice Care in America," pp. 370–71.

23. Ibid., p. 371.

24. World Health Organization, "The Global HIV/AIDS Situation," *A Point of Fact* (May 1991): 1–3.

3

The Hospice Approach to Medical Treatment for the Person with AIDS

Acquired Immunodeficiency Syndrome is a specific group of diseases or conditions which are indicative of severe immunosuppression related to infection with the human immunodeficiency virus (HIV). The case definition of AIDS was revised for surveillance purposes in August 1987, and is contained in the supplement of the *Morbidity and Mortality Weekly Report* published by the Centers for Disease Control in Atlanta, Georgia (1987). AIDS is defined there as an illness characterized by a list of "indicator" diseases, depending on the status of laboratory evidence of HIV infection. Some of the illnesses listed are candidiasis of the esophagus, trachea, bronchi, or lung; Kaposi's sarcoma (KS); Pneumocystis carinii pneumonia (PCP); cryptococcosis (a genus of yeastlike fungi); lymphoma of the brain; HIV wasting syndrome (emaciation); and HIV encephalopathy (brain disease).

Patients with HIV and AIDS may enjoy satisfactory health for

43

long periods. The median incubation period from infection with the virus to the development of AIDS has been estimated to be five years, but may be longer. Furthermore, even after a diagnosis of AIDS has been made, a person may live for several years.[1] Great progress has been made toward prolonging the lives of persons with AIDS, improving the quality of their lives, and alleviating suffering through a combination of scientific, clinical, and organizational expertise.[2] Internists and other specialists, who consult on HIV infected patients who are pregnant, have psychiatric symptoms, or require procedures for a non-AIDS related problem, are being encouraged to be vigilant in evaluating even minimal symptoms and signs. Patients who are susceptible to multiple disease processes that tend to be more severe than in otherwise healthy hosts, can be maintained in good health through preventive medicine.[3]

The goal of medical treatment during the final days or weeks of those with AIDS is to provide them with the optimal level of comfort through symptom and pain relief. Effective control of the physical symptoms must be tended to before all other needs are addressed.[4] That treatment is essential, since it helps avoid a long and painful dying that leaves the patient incapacitated; helpless; and without dignity, comfort, and human warmth. Those who administer the medical treatment need to reconcile themselves to the fact that there is no cure for AIDS and that even the most aggressive medical treatments are merely palliative since the underlying immunodeficiency remains.[5] Among the physical effects of AIDS are pain, pulmonary problems, gastrointestinal problems, genitourinary problems, skin problems, and fevers. Neuropsychological effects include AIDS dementia syndrome, depression, and delirium.

PAIN

Although comforting the sick has always been integral to medical treatment in general and to nursing in particular, the history of pain management is very short. Until the last twenty years, health care professionals in the United States did not focus on pain control and received inadequate training in this clinical area.[6] Pain was previously seen as a symptom to be eliminated by cure or control of its cause. Now, there is an effort to deal directly with pain itself, while a diagnosis or control is being established, or even when neither of those is possible. Research completed in the late 1960s and early 1970s showed that the patient was expected to suffer in silence. Later, the focus was placed on two types of programs in which pain relief was a top priority—childbirth education and hospice care.

The goal of pain management and intervention is to help the patient become pain-free or at least tolerate some pain at an acceptable level. The attending nurse must be able to assess the character and intensity of the pain and will then report these findings to the physician. Once a decision has been reached concerning the proper medication to use, careful consideration must be given to the route of administration of that medication. Because many persons with AIDS have major losses of muscle mass, it is difficult to find adequate tissue for intramuscular or hypodermic injections. Therefore, oral or intravenous routes of administration are the most effective. An underlying principle of management of pain attending chronic or acute disease is that it is far better to anticipate pain and give medication appropriately than to wait until the patient already has moderate or severe pain. In general, if this principle is followed, fewer analgesics will be needed over time.[7]

Regarding treatment of pain, it is conceptually useful to divide pain into two categories. Persons with AIDS experience pain that is due to a potentially reversible cause treatable by antibiotic therapy. There is also the pain whose cause is not directly treatable, either because maximum treatment has already been provided or because no direct treatment is at hand. It is this second category of pain which is the specific focus of palliative care. However, caregivers must always be careful not to overlook the pain that is directly treatable.[8]

Many AIDS patients complain of generalized discomfort that usually results from general debility, confinement to bed, or intermittent fevers causing aching muscles and joints. This nonspecific discomfort may be managed by general measures such as providing a comfortable mattress with foam pads or by gentle massage. When these measures are not sufficient, medications should be used.[9]

The pain may be linked to the multiple opportunistic diseases that afflict AIDS patients. For example, the pain may be related to the difficulty in breathing created by PCP and/or pulmonary Kaposi's sarcoma. It may result from enlarged lymph nodes. Anal pain may occur with herpes virus or other infections. Headaches may be caused by increased intracranial pressure from swelling of the brain or swelling that surrounds inflammatory mass lesions. Pain may also be due to the swelling that accompanies KS lesions in the groin that inhibit blood flow from the legs. In addition, painful skin breakdown may occur sometimes after radiation of the lesions. The resulting wounds are similar to pressure sores in their behavior and are often difficult to treat. Patients frequently experience pain on swallowing due to a yeast infection of the esophagus. Abdominal pain may be caused by several diseases. Finally, persons with AIDS often develop a painful peripheral neuropathy (a disease of the peripheral nerves) that decreases their ability to walk.[10,11]

Case Study

Even with the best of medical care, a person can suffer from a host of minor complaints that are not life-threatening, but which can make life unpleasant and at times unbearable.

"Peter," a health-care worker, underwent surgery for an inflamed appendix. Afterward, he did not recover; was unable to eat; and suffered from fever, weakness, and swollen lymph nodes. A test for AIDS came back positive. He subsequently became ill with a virus. Peter then had a bout with PCP and almost died. He also suffered from an itchy chest wall resulting from an attack of shingles, itchy feet due to a fungus that would not respond to local treatment and would not go away, oral and esophageal thrush, and warts on the face. The doctors were sympathetic, but were unable to offer him an acceptable level of relief.[12]

For mild or moderate pain, the first choice should be a medication such as acetaminophen (APAP) or a nonsteroidal anti-inflammatory drug (NSAID) that acts generally on the entire body. APAP is often the first choice because it is safe and has low incidence of side effects.

While the NSAIDs have proven to be more effective than APAP, there is a higher incidence of side effects. Aspirin (ASA) remains an excellent and inexpensive choice and relieves pain as effectively as APAP. ASA and other NSAIDs seem to be more effective fever-reducers, however.[13]

When pain is infrequent and intermittent, drugs are used on an as-needed basis. Pain relief will occur sooner but will be of shorter duration. Anti-inflammatory drugs such as ibuprofen, are commonly used. However, when the pain is persistent, an NSAID should be used at set time intervals. In this case, drugs whose effects last longer are recommended. In 6 percent to 10 percent of the patients, significant side effects (nausea, vomiting, upset stomach, and fluid retention) occur. Headaches result occasionally.[14]

In some cases, the peripherally acting pain reliever may be insufficient. A narcotic pain reliever that acts on the central nervous system (including the brain and spinal cord) is then added to APAP or NSAID. Codeine or its equivalent is often the first drug used, but some prefer to use oral morphine since it is reliable and has fewer side effects. Morphine has a low incidence of abuse by persons with AIDS because doses are easily adjusted; it provides about four hours of pain reduction. Many other effective narcotics are available. Longer-acting forms of morphine provide six to twelve hours of pain relief. Another choice, methadone, is effective and inexpensive.[15]

In order to prevent the pain associated with selected cases of terminal cancer, some patients have used a potent oral analgesic mixture known as Brompton's Cocktail, Brompton Mixture, or Hospice Mix. It normally contains a variable amount of morphine or diamorphine (heroin, in countries other than the United States), 10 milligrams of cocaine, 1.5 milliliters of ethyl alcohol (98 percent), 5 milliliters of flavoring syrup, and a variable amount of chloroform water. A mixture of morphine, cherry syrup, and a phenothiazine* has been used for years at Hospice, Inc., in New Haven, Connecticut.[16]

Proper use of the narcotic analgesic is more important than the specific choice. The correct dose, which is usually much higher than the dose needed to treat acute pain, is one that provides effective

---

*A group of chemically related compounds with various pharmacological actions

relief of pain. Loss of pain control results either from increased tolerance or disease progression. Increasing the dose of narcotics usually suffices to reestablish relief of pain.[17]

In AIDS patients, the pain from diseases of the peripheral nerves (usually causing weakness and numbness) and the intense pain felt at the site of a previous attack of shingles may not respond to narcotics alone. In some cases, amitriptyline has been helpful. This antidepressant has a mild tranquilizing action. If it is not sufficient, haloperidol, a tranquilizer used to relieve anxiety and tension, has been used successfully.

Persons with AIDS sometimes suffer pain when swallowing. To combat this pain, oral ketoconazole has been used for the fungal causes, while oral acyclovir has been used for pain caused by the herpes virus.

Headaches are common for AIDS patients and may be due to specific or nonspecific causes. Therapy can be initiated after a treatable pathogen is determined. In most cases, the pain is relieved through the treatment of the symptom. Oral steroids may be an option in this area.[18]

Finally, pain may be caused by an infection in both muscle and skin, especially when it occurs in the area around the rectum. Topical acyclovir may help, but oral therapy is usually required.[19]

PULMONARY PROBLEMS

Most persons with AIDS suffer from some form of pulmonary problem. Commonly seen problems include PCP, bacterial pneumonia or bronchitis, bronchospasm, viral pneumonia, pulmonary tuberculosis, or KS. Multiple problems may exist simultaneously.[20,21] Many AIDS patients are hospitalized due to PCP. About 50 percent of cases show PCP as the disease's first manifestation. Respiratory distress is characterized by wheezing, cough, shortness of breath, dyspnea (labored breathing) on exertion, tachypnea (rapid breathing), perspiration, and cyanosis (bluish or purplish discoloration).[22]

Frequent assessment of the respiratory status of the AIDS patient is absolutely essential. The primary goal in the treatment of patients suffering from respiratory distress is the achievement of an optimal level of comfort and ease in breathing. A secondary goal is the early discovery and treatment of infections of the respiratory tract.[23]

The treatment of infections of previously damaged lungs can provide the patient with some comfort. Two alternative in-hospital treatments for PCP are intravenous administration of trimethoprim-sulfamethoxazole, which prevents the growth of bacteria, or pentamidine.[24] Each treatment is similarly successful, in the range of 60 percent to 80 percent during initial episodes of PCP and somewhat less with subsequent infection. Both regimens have significant side effects, however, which often lead to their discontinuance. PCP can also be treated on an outpatient basis. Inhaled pentamidine (aerosolized via a nebulizer) is promising as an effective, relatively nontoxic therapy.[25]

As for treatment of the other pulmonary problems, oral antibiotics (erythromycin or amoxicillin) can be used to treat the patient with purulent sputum, especially if there are localized findings of rales* or pulmonary consolidation on exam. Bronchospasm may be alleviated by the use of drugs that are sprayed through metered dose inhalers, oral theophylline, or even oral steroids. Low-dose oral narcotics may be used to suppress coughs.[26] In most cases of deterioration of respiratory status, symptomatic treatment becomes the mainstay of pulmonary supportive care. The liberal use of oxygen is prescribed for dyspnea which can also be eased with oral morphine sulfate.[27]

GASTROINTESTINAL PROBLEMS

Several types of gastrointestinal problems may plague the AIDS patient. These conditions include oral problems, diarrhea, and nausea and vomiting.

First, there are oral problems that may cause much discomfort. Candida oropharyngitis can occur in the mouth as thrush, an infection of the tissues of the mouth that may appear as smooth, red, flat lesions or as creamy white patches. This disease can be painful, cause

---

*A soft, fine crackling sound heard in the lungs through a stethoscope

an unpleasant taste, and interfere with eating. Oral candidiasis can be treated in many ways. Nystatin can be taken orally as a liquid or by allowing nystatin tablets to dissolve in the mouth three times a day. Clotrimazole oral tablets are another option and may be more effective and convenient.[28] Mouthwashes, fizzy solutions, and flavored ice cubes may also be helpful.

Kaposi's sarcoma can cause infection or ulceration in the mouth and oropharynx. Obstructions of the airway or esophagus are the most significant complications. Other oral lesions include herpetic stomatitis (inflammation of the mucous membranes of the mouth), Herpes simplex lesions inside the mouth, Herpes zoster (shingles), severe Herpes zoster, severe periodontal disease, and hairy leuko-plakia, a white lesion appearing on the surface of the tongue.[29,30]

Another major problem is diarrhea, which is particularly trouble-some for the bedridden patient. More than 60 percent of AIDS patients suffer from this. Diarrhea may result from infections that are treatable (Shigella, Salmonella, Campylobacter, Giardia lamblia, and E. histo-lytica) or from infections that do not respond to specific treatment (Cryptoporidium, Isopora, and mycobacterium avium intracellulare [MAI]). For symptomatic treatment of diarrhea, nonprescription remedies (Kaopectate® or Pepto Bismol®) or bulk are rarely effective. Diphenoxylate hydrochloride tablets or liquid, or loperamide may be helpful. If not, oral narcotics may be necessary.[31]

If the diarrhea persists, all that can be hoped for is a slowing of the condition. This is often the case when KS is the cause. In this situation, the goal of medical care is to provide adequate nutrition and hydration to help the patient retain good circulation. The patient's weight, intake and output of solids and liquids, caloric intake, and electrolytes (the concentration of separate ions in the blood) should be monitored.

AIDS patients often suffer from nausea and vomiting. Since nausea can be caused by many medications, it is important to review the current medications and discontinue those that are no longer necessary or are marginally beneficial. Other possible sources of nausea and vomiting are systemic infection, adrenal insufficiency, hyper-calcemia (an abnormally high rate of calcium deposits in the blood), kidney or liver failure, inflammation of the esophagus, or fecal impaction (hardened feces in the rectum or colon, often requiring surgical removal).[32,33] If a specific cause cannot be uncovered, then symptomatic treatment is necessary. Prochlorperazine is usually effective; however, if this drug fails, then alternative selection of medications should be based on receptor site theory, which involves selecting medications on the basis of the receptors* that need to be blocked.[34]

GENITOURINARY PROBLEMS

Urinary incontinence or retention are also common problems for the person with AIDS. While these conditions are normally of neurological origin, they may also be due to medication side effects or infection.[35,36] Retention and incontinence may both be treated with a catheter or an intermittent catheterization program.[37]

SKIN PROBLEMS

As a result of weight loss and emaciation, patients usually experience alteration in the passage of fluid through tissue and/or significant loss of muscle mass, which leads to skin breakdown. The prevention, minimization, and healing of pressure sores are the main goals for skin care. The nurse should examine the patient's skin condition, particularly in the areas of the bony prominences and assess and document reddened skin, pain, numbness, and blisters. Frequent position changes and maintenance of body alignment are important. A kinetic air bed may be considered for prevention of pressure sores. Mobility should be encouraged as activity is the key to prevention of skin breakdown.[38] Baths, showers, and gentle massaging with an oily preparation also have great therapeutic value for skin care.

---

*A receptor is a specialized cell or tissue sensitive to a specific stimulus, e.g., a sensory nerve ending or sense organ.

FEVERS

Fevers in AIDS patients may be a sign of infection or evidence of a treatment failure in a patient who was previously without a fever. They can also be caused by chemotherapy.[39] A combination of therapies may be used to help the patient avoid fever. Acetaminophin, tepid or alcohol baths, and/or a cooling blanket may be needed. Since insensible water losses occur during the fevers and the "sweats," fluid intake must be monitored.[40]

AIDS DEMENTIA SYNDROME

As many as 65 percent of persons with AIDS suffer from dementia, which is a loss of intellectual capabilities associated with impairment of memory and higher cortical function occurring in the brain. The early symptoms are cognitive (forgetfulness, inability to concentrate, confusion, and/or slowness of thought), motor (loss of balance, weakness, or deterioration in other skills), and behavioral (apathy, withdrawal, and mood change, including psychosis). The symptoms may be very mild, accompanied by only small changes in personality and initially may be attributed to anxiety or depression, or to a patient's awareness of physical deterioration. It may be difficult to distinguish dementia from other causes of change in personality. For an accurate diagnosis, mental testing is needed. Early and accurate diagnosis is important to put changes in perspective and prepare for future needs. Dementia can initially appear as functional psychological disorders such as depression, anxiety, panic attacks, paranoia, bipolar episodes,* or even schizophrenia.[41]

The course of deterioration varies from patient to patient. Dementia progresses slowly in some patients while in others, deterioration is observed over a period of months. Patients usually become incapable of caring for themselves and require twenty-four-hour care and supervision.

AIDS dementia has many causes, several of which may coexist

---

*A disorder characterized by both manic and depressive episodes in an individual patient. The most common cause of this form of dementia is presumed to be direct involvement of the brain by the AIDS virus. Patients may also have vision problems, seizures, muscle twitching, or weakness or numbness in the nerves. Other causes of dementia in AIDS include lymphoma of the brain, cryptococcosis, cerebral bleeding or dead tissue due to lack of blood, and rarely candiadiasis, aspergillosis (fungus in the tissues or mucous membranes), histoplasmosis (a pulmonary infection caused by mold), and severe vitamin deficiency. Most of the causes are not treatable. However, toxoplasmosis, which can cause dementia, can be diagnosed through magnetic resonance imaging, which demonstrates a mass lesion. Therapy with drugs used in chemotherapy, such as sulfadiazine, pyrimethamine, and leucovorin, can often shrink the lesions. Finally, dementia may be caused or accelerated by narcotics, sedative-hypnotics, and antidepressants. Concurrent physical problems such as systemic infection, hypoxia (subnormal levels of oxygen in blood and tissue), fluid or electrolyte disturbances, and anemia may accelerate dementia as well.[42,43]

The mainstays of treatment are psychosocial and environmental approaches. A large calendar and a clock in conspicuous places are orienting cues. The patient should be made aware of all appointments and scheduled visitors. Names of caregivers and important phone numbers should be easily accessible. Every effort must be made to help the patient compensate for the effects of dementia. In addition, medications may be necessary to assist the patient in coping with sleeplessness, emotional instability, hallucinations, suspiciousness, and agitation. Medications such as haloperidol and lorazepam may help control anxiety and some of the other problems, but drugs affecting the central nervous system should be used at the lowest possible doses.[44]

DEPRESSION

Many AIDS patients suffer a loss of self-esteem, experience feelings of failure, lose interest in people, have intense guilt feelings or suicidal thoughts, and suffer from frequent crying spells. The caregiver must focus on these cognitive and affective symptoms of depression, not on the involuntary bodily signs.[45,46] For the treatment of depression, low doses of amitriptyline or doxepin have been helpful. Counseling should be an adjunct to the use of medications, since people who are dying have to cope with the emotional effects of the diagnosis of terminal disease, progressive physical deterioration, psychosocial changes, and progressive loss of capacity.[47]

DELIRIUM

Delirium may be seen at any stage of AIDS and may be misdiagnosed as depression or some other psychiatric disorder. It may be caused by infection, hypoxia (an oxygen deficiency in the tissues), or electrolyte imbalance coupled with psychological distress, isolation, sleep disturbance, and sensory deprivation. Delirium's hallmarks are an intermittent clouding of consciousness along with cognitive dysfunction. Anti-psychotic or anti-anxiety medications such as haloperidol or lorazepam are often useful for the treatment of delirium.[48,49]

CONCLUSION

Although significant progress has been made toward prolonging the lives of persons with AIDS, the sad truth is that AIDS is relentless and inevitably fatal. However, there is often an incubation period between the time of diagnosis with HIV and the onset of AIDS. Once AIDS has been diagnosed, the persons with AIDS may be faced with a number of medical conditions including pain, pulmonary problems, gastrointestinal problems, genitourinary problems, skin problems, and fevers. The hospice approach seeks to alleviate these symptoms. Medical treatment is focused on providing the patient with as much comfort as possible through symptom and pain relief.

While this chapter has focused on the manner in which medical treatment attempts to maintain a high quality of life in terminal AIDS patients, a word about the role of health professionals in the lives of those who are HIV seronegative is important. People who have been told that they are infected with HIV are often condemned to an agonizing period of anticipatory anxiety before actual disease symptoms occur. They suffer from "symptoms of awareness," resulting from the fear and anxiety induced by the knowledge that they are infected. The primary manifestation of this state is the preoccupation with minor complaints. Physicians and caregivers, while remaining understanding, must emphasize the positive aspects of the patient's present state of objective good health.[50]

The hospice approach to medical treatment of the problems that a person with AIDS may encounter can be very beneficial. Hospice centers not only on the disease itself, but also on patients and their families. The hospice program emphasizes the well-being of the family unit and adapts the care to meet varied individual needs. As patients face death, comfort, care, and support are provided. Hospice focuses on the quality of life and on making the dying process as comfortable as possible for both patients and their loved ones.

NOTES

1. M. W. Adler, "Care for Patients with HIV Infection and AIDS," *British Medical Journal* 295 (1987): 29.

2. G. H. Friedland, "Clinical Care in the AIDS Epidemic," *Daedalus* 118 (1989): 61–62.

3. B. Feinman and A. E. Glatt, "General Medical Consultation of the Patient with HIV Infection," *Journal of Palliative Care* 4 (1988): 37.

4. The Expert Working Group on Integrated Palliative Care for Persons with AIDS, "Caring Together: Summary of a report submitted to Health and Welfare Canada," *Journal of Palliative Care* 4 (1987): 76–86.

5. C. Clark, et al., "Hospice Care: A Model for Caring for the Person with AIDS," *Nursing Clinics of North America* 23 (1988): 852.

6. M. McCaffery, "Pain Management: Nurses Lead the Way to New Priorities," *American Journal of Nursing* 90 (1990): 45–47.

7. J. D. Durham and F. L. Cohen, *The Person with AIDS: Nursing Perspectives* (New York: Springer Publishing Co., 1987), p. 98.

8. J. Schoefferman, "Pain: Diagnosis and Management in the Palliative Control of AIDS," *Journal of Palliative Care* 4 (1988): 46.

9. J. Schoefferman, "Care of the AIDS Patient," *Death Studies* 12 (1988): 435–36.

10. Durham and Cohen, *The Person with AIDS,* p. 98.

11. J. Schoefferman, "Hospice Care of the Patient with AIDS," *The Hospice Journal* 3 (1987): 60–61.

12. P. Phoenix, "Alive with AIDS," in *Living with AIDS,* S. R. Graubard, ed. (Cambridge, Mass.: The MIT Press, 1990), pp. 151–58.

13. J. Schoefferman, "Care of the AIDS Patient," pp. 438–39.

14. Ibid.

15. Ibid., p. 436.

16. K. P. Cohen, *Hospice, Prescription for Terminal Care* (Germantown, Md.: Aspen Systems Corporation, 1979), p. 96.

17. Schoefferman, "Care of the AIDS Patient," p. 436.

18. Ibid., p. 437.

19. Ibid.

20. Ibid., pp. 438–39.

21. Schoefferman, "Hospice Care of the Patient with AIDS," pp. 61–63.

22. Durham and Cohen, *The Person with AIDS,* pp. 101–103.

23. Ibid.

24. Schoefferman, "Care of the AIDS Patient," pp. 438–39.

25. G. Friedberg and A. E. Glatt, "Management of AIDS-Related Infections with an Accent on Outpatient Therapy and Prophylaxis," *Journal of Palliative Care* 4 (1988): 39.

26. Schoefferman, "Care of the AIDS Patient," pp. 438–39.

27. Schoefferman, "Hospice Care of the Patient with AIDS," p. 62.

28. Schoefferman, "Care of the AIDS Patient," p. 439.

29. Ibid., pp. 439–40.

30. Schoefferman, "Hospice Care of the Patient with AIDS," pp. 63–65.

31. Schoefferman, "Care of the AIDS Patient," p. 440.

32. Ibid., pp. 439–40.

33. Schoefferman, "Hospice Care of the Patient with AIDS," pp. 63–65.

34. Schoefferman, "Care of the AIDS Patient," pp. 440–41.

35. Ibid.

36. Schoefferman, "Hospice Care of the Patient with AIDS," pp. 65–66.

37. Schoefferman, "Care of the AIDS Patient," p. 441.

38. Durham and Cohen, *The Person with AIDS,* pp. 104–105.

39. Ibid.

40. Ibid., pp. 105–107.

41. Schoefferman, "Care of the AIDS Patient," pp. 441–45.

42. Ibid.

43. Schoefferman, "Hospice Care of the Patient with AIDS," pp. 66–68.

44. Schoefferman, "Care of the AIDS Patient," pp. 442–43.

45. Ibid., pp. 441–45.

46. Schoefferman, "Hospice Care of the Patient with AIDS," pp. 66–68.

47. Schoefferman, "Care of the AIDS Patient," pp. 442–43.

48. Ibid., pp. 441–45.

49. Schoefferman, "Hospice Care of the Patient with AIDS," pp. 60–61.

50. D. K. MacFadden, "Symptom Control in AIDS," *Journal of Palliative Care* 4 (1988): 42–43.

4

Emotional and Social Issues Related to Hospice Care for the Person with AIDS

Fear and AIDS run hand-in-hand. People are afraid of contracting the virus. Many thought that they were safe if they did not participate in any "risk-taking" behaviors. Now, however, other issues have been brought to the surface regarding HIV. Health care workers, patients, physicians, and all other types of people are concerned. To settle some of these fears and to gain a better understanding of the issues, knowledge and education are needed.

Along with hospice and AIDS come many issues that need to be considered. The physicians' attitudes toward hospice are important, especially if they resist the concept. Health care workers' attitudes and ideas about persons with AIDS (PWAs) are very relevant. Another major issue is the screening of health care workers for HIV. The role of both palliative and aggressive care in the hospice program and decision making for the continuance of care are two matters that often arise. And finally, the quality of life needs to be evaluated in both hospice and nonhospice settings.

PHYSICIANS' ATTITUDES TOWARD HOSPICE

Physicians are sometimes resistant to the concept of hospice. One reason underlying this resistance is the physician's own attitude toward death. A study comparing physicians' fears of death with the fears of healthy and seriously (some terminally) ill patients revealed that physicians showed significantly more fear of death than either the healthy or sick lay people. While this fear seems today to be a factor in certain physicians' selection of medicine as a career—modern medicine being looked on as an aggressive *conquest* of death—it also may prevent them from being able to help patients deal with impending death.[1]

The physician's discomfort in this area of patient support is of relatively recent origin. Until forty years ago, cure was rare, and death was accepted as a natural consequence of having lived. The primary obligation of the physician was to bring comfort to the patient, whether that patient was going to get better or not. Now that medical science has learned how to cure far more effectively, death has come to be seen as unnatural and as the enemy of the physician.[2] Supported by the advanced medical training that has been in place since after World War II, as well as by the arsenal of antibiotics and other interventions, most physicians believe that they can cure most diseases. They forget that most serious illness in this society results from chronic and not acute disease, and is therefore not amenable to seemingly magical technical interventions. They believe overwhelmingly that the goal of their endeavors should be to cure and that anything less is failure.[3]

Another reason for some physicians' resistance to hospice is that they see it primarily as a nursing function: a system of giving care rather than prescribing cure. When investigation, diagnosis, prolongation of life, and cure no longer seem relevant, physicians seem to conclude that they have nothing more to offer and therefore tend to remove themselves from the picture. However, a great deal remains for physicians to do for the dying person once cure is no longer a possibility.[4] They can help the patient cope with the frightening experience of the dying process. Patients fear the indignity of bodily degeneration, which includes loss of bowel control, offensive odors, disfiguring lesions, dependence on others, pain, suffocation, dementia, and abandonment. Competent and caring physicians can explain the course of the illness clearly to patients and can anticipate problems to allow for early intervention. They can also assist patients in gaining some measure of control over their lives by teaching them the proper use of medications and other ways to remain in charge of their health.[5]

More and more physicians are referring PWAs to hospice programs. While this is often an appropriate action, there is a potential danger that their frustration with being unable to cure these persons may lead them to make the referral too soon.[6]

ATTITUDE OF HEALTH CARE WORKERS TOWARD PWAS

Working with persons with AIDS presents many difficulties for health care workers. First of all, since those suffering from the disease are mostly young men and women in their thirties and forties, young doctors and nurses have to deal with the issue of identifying and coming to terms with their own vulnerability and mortality. For physicians in particular, this compounds their great fear of death.

Fear of transmission of the deadly disease is also common among health care workers. While the risk is low and measures exist to further reduce that risk, accidental injury and infection is certainly possible.[7] In the summer of 1987, the Centers for Disease Control (CDC) indicated that three health care workers who were splashed with HIV seropositive blood became infected with HIV. This manner of exposure was not previously thought to be a hazard. Other researchers demonstrated that occupational transmission of HIV would not be limited to being accidentally stuck with AIDS-infected needles. Consequently, health care workers began to file suits; furthermore, physicians and other health care workers began refusing surgery to PWAs and limiting the care they might receive. As a result of this fear on the part of the health community, HIV seropositive individuals may now have difficulty receiving the medical attention they need.

Health administrators must be sensitive to the fears of the health care workers in their institutions. It is not helpful to cite statistics to an individual who has slashed his hand while doing a spinal tap on a woman with a history of IV-drug use or to someone else who is experiencing symptoms that might be AIDS-related. Administrators should also ensure that they are following all recommended procedures for the protection of their workers. Even so, workers' professional and moral obligations toward the patients they serve must be made clear to them.

Health care professionals may have difficulty treating AIDS patients with respect, because AIDS has been considered by many to be a "dirty disease" contracted by homosexuals and intravenous drug users, who for many are pariahs in this society. Many people believe that persons with AIDS have brought the infection on themselves; therefore, they do not deserve compassion. Others tend to classify AIDS cases as either "innocent" victims (such as infants, hemophiliacs, and transfusion recipients) or "guilty" victims (including IV-drug users and homosexuals).[8] It is difficult for health care workers to escape society's prejudices. Society at large condemns homosexuality and fails to come to terms with the nature of addiction. Because many of the addicted turn to crime to support their habits, addiction becomes synonymous with criminality in the eyes of many.

Case Study

A twenty-nine-year-old man with severe classic hemophilia came to a local hospital because he felt very dizzy and fainted each time he stood. The hospital knew him will since he had a seven-year history of HIV infection and AIDS-related syndromes. The emergency room triage nurse determined that this was not an emergency and left him waiting in the waiting room for four hours. The patient, not having the physical strength to protest, was finally seen by an intern. Even though the patient was severely anemic, the intern delayed treatment for at least an hour after having examined him. The resident in charge of the emergency room knew the patient had low blood pressure and was a hemophiliac, but did not treat him as a critically ill case.

Ordinarily that patient's symptoms would be suggestive of a gastrointestinal hemorrhage, yet no attempts were made to consider treating the bleeding diathesis early on. Perhaps, consciously or subconsciously, this competent and energetic team decided to treat this patient differently because he had AIDS.[9]

SCREENING OF HEALTH CARE WORKERS

The public's fear of being infected by a seropositive caregiver has been an issue for some time now. This fear has led some to demand that health care workers be tested. In August 1987, the CDC stated that up to that point, there had been no reports of transmission of HIV from infected health care workers to patients. It did point out, however, that transmission during invasive procedures remained a possibility.[10] A recent investigation by the CDC found it likely that a Florida dentist, Dr. David J. Acer of Stuart, had transmitted HIV to three of his patients. The dentist has since died.[11] Among the more than 160,000 cases of AIDS reported since the initial outbreak in 1981, these are the only known incidents of probable transmission from a health care worker to a patient.

Many questions are raised by this issue. Among the more crucial questions arising is, Should caregivers be tested? In closing a two-day meeting that discussed the risk of transmission of HIV from doctors and dentists to their patients, Dr. William Roper, head of the CDC, affirmed that, in the opinion of most, the mandatory testing of health care workers for AIDS was neither necessary or useful. (He did not, however, discuss whether health care workers already infected with AIDS should be required to inform their patients.) The consensus at the meeting focused on the need for greater application of infection-control procedures and continued research to develop better and safer equipment in order to protect both patients and health care workers, including the issuance of new guidelines to protect patients against transmission of the AIDS virus from health care workers.[12]

The wisdom of mandatory testing of all health care workers does indeed seem questionable. While it is true that three patients seem to have been infected by a health care worker, this rare occurrence cannot be used to justify the invasive and costly enterprise such a testing program would involve. And while transmission of the hepatitis

B virus (HBV), a blood-borne agent with a considerably greater potential for spread from health care workers to patients, has been documented, that mode of infection has occurred only during the performance of certain types of invasive procedures. Strict adherence to infection-control measures will result in minimal risk of transmission. If such testing is ever put in place, the same principles of testing that are used in testing programs of patients should govern this program. Those principles are:

(1) Consent should be obtained.

(2) The worker must be informed of the results and counseling must be provided for that person.

(3) Confidentiality must be assured so that the knowledge is limited to those with a need to know.

(4) There must be an evaluation of the efficacy of the program in reducing the incidence of infection of patients by health care providers and of the effect of the procedure on the health care worker.[13]

A serious consideration of the fourth principle might lead to the conclusion that such a program is not useful or cost-effective.

The question remains: Should health care providers who are seropositive be allowed to practice, or should they be discharged or limited in their practice? Since health care institutions have not formulated a stable policy, the relatively few employees whose cases have come to the institution's (and the public's) attention have been dealt with on a case-to-case basis.[14] Some fear that the new guidelines to be issued by the CDC could include proposals to restrict the practice of infected health care workers.[15] Such restrictions can only exacerbate the epidemic of fear already existing in the community; furthermore, they may distract the medical community from the efforts it must make for infection control. And finally, such regulations would protect no one. The identified seropositive person would be restricted, while unidentified health care workers would be practicing without restriction. Such restrictions may impact on the health system with a deadly irony: they may effectively reduce the number of individuals willing to work with AIDS patients, since these restrictions would in effect eliminate from the field of clinical practice the very caregivers who might be most sympathetic to persons with AIDS. This would worsen an already serious shortage of health care workers available to provide necessary services to people with AIDS.[16]

PALLIATIVE CARE VERSUS AGGRESSIVE CARE

Should aggressive care be used in a hospice setting? With the hope for a cure being ever present, there may exist an ambivalent attitude toward relinquishing treatment. Persons with AIDS often seek palliative therapy while simultaneously seeking curative therapy. On-going discussion between patient, physician, nurse, and other team members is vital and should include when to stop curative therapy. The family, who is considered the unit of care, should also be involved in these discussions. However, the patient must be considered the key member of the team, deciding preferences for treatment, home or hospital management, and type and number of social interactions.[17]

Even in the terminal phases, active interventions may be appropriate in some cases. One example is the early use of ganeyelovir to prevent blindness resulting from retinitis caused by a herpes virus. The positive result of this therapy must be weighed against the trauma that accompanies this kind of treatment. The patient must have a central line inserted and have infusions two times per day for two weeks followed thereafter by infusions daily or several times a week. This curative therapy may be chosen by the patient either on his own or following consultation with members of the team. While all team members should provide their honest input, the final decision should be left to the patient.[18]

Persons with AIDS who dread the onset of HIV encephalopathy (brain disease) have the possibility of taking oral zidovudine, consequently adding to the quality of their lives. Some patients may choose to forego this active therapy because of the trauma of the regular blood transfusions that are often required.[19] While tests have shown that zidovudine may extend a patient's life for more than a year,[20] the patient will have to make the decision whether the extra time gained by the treatment justifies the steps he or she has to take to extend that life.

In the final analysis, while aggressive care may be appropriate in some instances for persons with AIDS in a hospice program, only palliative care is ultimately relevant.[21]

Case Studies

The first case illustrates the moment of decision in the life of a patient whose life was being extended by blood transfusions. "Jim" had suffered from AIDS for thirteen months and was in the last stages of the disease. He had had one devastating onslaught of Pneumocystis pneumonia and was thought to have Kaposi's sarcoma (KS) lesions in his esophagus, making swallowing very difficult. The physician believed that these lesions were causing the steady fall in Jim's blood count. Yet blood transfusions no longer produced any noticeable improvement in his energy level. On the day Jim died, he had requested one more unit of red blood cells to give him energy over the weekend. While waiting for the blood to arrive, he became increasingly nauseated and weak, and vomited three cups of fresh blood, indicating an acute gastrointestinal bleeding. He and his hospice nurse discussed his next course of action. The hospice nurse told him he would most likely die in the next few hours if he did not go to the hospital for treatment of the active bleeding. He decided not to seek treatment and died that evening with his family and pastor at his bedside.[22]

The second case history is that of a thirty-five-year-old married mother of two children, employed as a secretary. She was diagnosed with an advanced malignant tumor of the upper chest wall and armpit with the presumed primary location of the cancer to have been in the breast. Two months later, the social worker from the palliative care team met her on an initial visit to the outpatient oncology clinic. The involvement of a member of the palliative care team at a point far before the terminal stage of illness allowed the professional caregivers to help her until she died. It also supported her right to make "care-or-cure" choices. The social worker helped not only the couple, but also their children in exploring how seriously ill the patient was. As her condition deteriorated, the various therapies that were attempted failed. The patient had uncontrollable movement of her left arm, unceasing nausea and vomiting, and poor pain control. She had numerous medical interventions during her hospital stay. Decisions concerning those interventions were made through ongoing discussions between the patient, family, palliative care team, family physician, nursing staff, resident physicians, consultants, and housekeepers.

The team decided that it would be flexible as an interdisciplinary health service delivery team. Although some of her choices for intervention seemed inappropriate to the palliative care team and others appeared poor choices to the oncology team, everyone supported her right to make those decisions. They included the patient's remaining in the hospital when she was physically able to be home, and her choosing which drugs to take for relief of symptoms and which blood tests to have. The group supported her when she brought in outside drugs and herbal cures.

A week before she died, the patient was angry "that there were no treatments left." She managed all her medications, including ones for pain. Only on the morning of her death did she release management of her treatment plan and allow the team to decide what was best for her. The team had acted in this way because they wanted to give her the choice to live her own life until she died.[23]

DECISION MAKING FOR CONTINUANCE OF CARE

Another issue to be discussed is the decision about responding to an "untreatable condition" such as respiratory failure. Who will make the decision whether or not to put the patient on a life-support system? This issue is particularly difficult in cases where the person with AIDS is no longer competent because of a neuropsychological condition. If the unit of palliative care is the family, who should be considered "family"? If the AIDS patient is living with a lover, who can make this type of decision in the absence of a durable power of attorney?[24]

It seems that the right time to reach these decisions is early on in the course of the disease, when the patient is capable of participating. A "living will" should be considered; however, this is not done in many cases, since health care givers are reluctant to discuss such an issue with new patients when they are still well. The problem is compounded by the fact that the patient population is young (average age twenty-eight to thirty-four), highly intelligent (with an average length of sixteen years of formal education in the first 10,000 U.S. cases), and often from strongly artistic backgrounds. Young women and children are also affected. It is difficult or impossible to discuss this kind of issue with what some care givers consider "sympathetic" victims such as hemophiliacs, blood transfusion-related cases, and babies. All these factors make discussion about the future course of treatment problematic.[25]

Case Study

"Frank" was a thirty-six-year-old man who was told by his doctor that he suspected Frank had AIDS after he had complained of specific symptoms—fatigue for about six months, diarrhea for four weeks, and some difficulty with concentration. Frank had admitted to his family physician that he was gay and that he had had a stable five-year relationship with Bill. Frank was ultimately diagnosed with Pneumocystis pneumonia. Further testing showed moderate cognitive impairment. When the hospital decided that more tests were necessary, they were not sure who was empowered to give consent to the planned investigations. Frank himself was unable to give informed consent at that point.

Frank's parents, Susan and Paul, aware of their son's sexual orientation, had had little contact with him over the past few years. When the medical team contacted Susan and Paul, they appeared at the ward, nearly in shock, and gave consent for further testing. There followed discussion of who would care for Frank now that he could not care for himself. Although Bill insisted that he and Frank had agreed that Bill would care for him, there was no documentation to support Bill's position.

Frank's parents insisted that they should take care of their son in his last days. Frank was unable to express any clear thoughts over this matter. The only sign of his intention was when he moved his chair close to Bill during one of the discussions. The palliative care physician, who met with all of them, helped them reach a mutually acceptable decision. Frank would stay with Bill in their apartment. Susan and Paul would provide some help in looking after Frank two or three days a week while Bill went to work to look after his business. Frank was subsequently hospitalized on two occasions. He died peacefully at home three months later.[26]

QUALITY OF LIFE: HOSPICE VERSUS NONHOSPICE CARE

Does hospice as a model of terminal care achieve the outcomes claimed by its proponents? Is there a difference between hospice and non-hospice patients' quality of life? According to a comprehensive survey of literature on this issue made by Vincent Mor, the dimensions of quality of life that were measured in various studies included: pain, symptoms, and physical quality of life; satisfaction with care; patients' psychosocial outcomes; where patients die; and family members outcomes, both psychosocial and health-related. Let us examine these factors individually.

The studies showed that hospice clearly does not result in patients experiencing increased pain. In fact, some comparisons report that hospice may achieve small but significant differences in pain control. The differences were observable only when the base rates of pain in the study population were relatively high and when information was received from observers rather than from the patients since they were often too sick to report on their own condition.[27]

Hospice claims that the severity of symptoms, such as difficulty in breathing, nausea, and vomiting, as well as indicators of cognitive functioning, might be affected by hospice. The results in the literature concerning the comparison of the level of symptoms in hospice and nonhospice patients were mixed. There were also varying results concerning the level of cognitive functioning. There is still insufficient evidence that hospice is more effective than conventional care in controlling patients' physical symptoms and maintaining patients' awareness of their surroundings.[28]

Overall quality of life refers to both physical and psychosocial functioning. The studies concluded that quality of life relating to physical functioning does not appear to be affected, either for good or ill, by hospice. Those findings concerning psychosocial functioning were even more ambiguous.[29]

Patients served in hospices were more satisfied, overall, with the care that they received than nonhospice patients. This positive effect, however, may be associated only with the inpatient variety of hospice. The studies also found that although the families of home care patients were satisfied, they were not significantly more satisfied than were nonhospice patients' families. In general, however, hospice does appear to provide to the patients and the families the kind of service that they want. They have fewer regrets about the orientation of the care received than do nonhospice patients.[30]

The studies focusing on patient psychosocial outcomes seem to indicate that the hospice philosophy does not have the indirect effect on the patients' psychological status at which hospice aims. The evidence suggests that explicit psychosocial intervention can work, at least under optimal conditions. The problem in the ultimate analysis may be financial. Will these programs be able to pay for the integration of psychosocial and medical services?[31]

Hospice does facilitate arrangements for dying at home for those patients and families desiring it, whereas the nonhospice system does not. There were differences in the likelihood of death at home between the hospice program emphasizing home care and the hospices with inpatient units. In the program that emphasized home care, between 30 percent and 70 percent of patients died at home. In the inpatient units, between 20 percent and 30 percent did. The hospice movement allows for choice, since death at home is not necessarily to be desired in all cases.[32]

Studies of the impact of the program on the family's anxiety and depression while the patient was living produced contradictory findings. One study found primary care persons in hospital-based hospices to be more satisfied with the care than primary care persons in conventional care situations. This may be due to hospice families feeling more involved in the care. In a home care setting, however, the involvement often becomes so intense that the family ends up feeling burdened.[33]

Bereavement affects people's health. Indeed, the grief of bereavement can seriously affect those with preexisting health problems. Studies of the effects of hospice bereavement counseling has resulted in mixed findings, which may be due to the fact that a high proportion of people not really in need of counseling were included in the studies. Also, every hospice defines bereavement services differently. The literature seems to indicate that only a minority of bereaved persons can benefit from intervention. It also appears that the most effective programs are those that are professionally administered with interpersonal contact over several months and those that are targeted only to the people who really need the counseling.[34]

CONCLUSION

This chapter has discussed the issues of the physician's attitudes toward hospice, the attitudes of health care workers toward those suffering from AIDS, screening of health care workers for AIDS, the relationship between curative and palliative care, the determination of who should make decisions for persons with AIDS when they are no longer capable of making decisions for themselves due to neuropsychological problems, and the comparative quality of care for the terminally ill in hospice and nonhospice settings. While all these issues are important, perhaps the most crucial are the attitudes of health care workers toward hospice and toward people with AIDS, and the necessity for the administration and staff in hospice programs constantly to reevaluate the ways in which they implement the philosophy of care to which they are dedicated. Unless more health care workers are willing to participate in programs that serve AIDS patients, there will not be a sufficient number of workers to maintain these programs at a proper level of care. Also, the goals toward which the advocates of the hospice philosophy work can be more effectively attained only through constant evaluation of their programs. These evaluations, coupled with critical thinking, may serve as a guide to them in considering future directions.

In the future, many more people will be exposed to AIDS. The exposure may be physical, emotional, and/or social. Only through knowledge and understanding will people's fears decrease. Because of this, education and awareness pertaining to hospice and AIDS issues is of the utmost importance.

NOTES

1. R. W. Buckingham, *Care of the Dying Child: A Practical Guide for Those Who Help Others* (New York: Continuum, 1990), p. 23.

2. W. Bulkin and H. Lukashok, "Rx for Dying: The Case for Hospice," *The New England Journal of Medicine* 318 (1988): 376–78.

3. G. H. Friedland, "Clinical Care in the AIDS Epidemic," *Daedalus* 118 (1989): 70–71.

4. Bulkin and Lukashok, "Rx for Dying: The Case for Hospice," p. 377.

5. J. Schoefferman, "Care of the AIDS Patient," *Death Studies* 12 (1988): 446.

6. Bulkin and Lukashok, "Rx for Dying: The Case for Hospice," p. 377.

7. Friedland, "Clinical Care in the AIDS Epidemic," pp. 67–68.

8. Ibid., p. 69.

9. C. M. Tsoukas, "The Dying Leper Syndrome," *Journal of Palliative Care* 4 (1988): 13–14.

10. U.S. Department of Health and Human Services, Centers for Disease Control. Morbidity and Mortality Weekly Report (Supplement). *Review of the CDC Surveillances Case Definition for Acquired Immunodeficiency Syndrome,* 36, 1S (1987): 15.

11. L. K. Altman, "AIDS Tests of Health Workers Called Unnecessary," *The New York Times,* February 23, 1991, p. 9.

12. Ibid.

13. U.S. Department of Health and Human Services, Centers for Disease Control. Morbidity and Mortality Weekly Report. *Recommendations for Prevention of HIV Transmission in Health Care Settings,* 36, 2S (1987): 15-S.

14. Institute of Medicine, National Academy of Sciences, *Confronting AIDS: Update 1988* (Washington, D.C.: National Academy Press, 1988), p. 100.

15. L. K. Altman, "AIDS Tests of Health Workers Called Unnecessary," *The New York Times,* February 23, 1991, p. 9.

16. Friedland, "Clinical Care in the AIDS Epidemic," pp. 77–78.

17. C. Clark, A. Curley, A. Hughes, and R. James, "Hospice Care: A Model for Caring for the Persons with AIDS," *Nursing Clinics of North America* 23 (1988): 852.

18. V. Moss, "The Mildmay Approach," *Journal of Palliative Care* 4 (1988): 105.

19. Ibid.

20. W. A. Haseltine, "Prospects for the Medical Control of the AIDS Epidemic," *Daedalus* 118 (1989): 14.

21. Bulkin and Lukashok, "Rx for Dying: The Case for Hospice," p. 377.

22. H. Anderson and P. MacElveen-Hoehn, "Gay Clients with AIDS: New Challenges for Hospice Programs," *The Hospice Journal* 4 (1988): 38–39.

23. J. A. O'Connor, F. I. Burge, B. T. King, and J. Epstein, "Does Care Exclude Cure in Palliative Care?" *Journal of Palliative Care* 2 (1986): 11–15.

24. P. W. A. Mansell, "AIDS: Home, Ambulatory, and Palliative Care," *Journal of Palliative Care* 4 (1988): 31–32.

25. Ibid.

26. S. L. Librach, "Who's in Control? What's in a Family?" *Journal of Palliative Care* 4 (1988): 11–12.

27. V. Mor, *Hospice Care Systems: Structure, Process, Costs, and Outcome* (New York: Springer Publications, 1987), p. 140.

28. Ibid., p. 141.

29. Ibid., p. 142.

30. Ibid., p. 156.

31. Ibid., p. 166.

32. Ibid., p. 150.

33. Ibid., p. 168.

34. Ibid., p. 176.

5

How to Develop Hospice Programs
for Persons with AIDS

CARES AND CONCERNS

The care of the acutely ill person with AIDS requires the most skillful application of nursing knowledge.[1] Many of the quidelines for the care of patients with AIDS parallel those for the patients who present with other pulmonary, neurologic, oncologic, and systemic diseases.[2] However, unlike these patients, persons with AIDS often experience more adverse reactions to medications and present special challenges because of lifestyle issues related to their diseases and care.[3] When caring for people with AIDS, one must realize that they are carrying a lot of "baggage," including rejection, isolation, hostility, depression, denial, and anger. Those working with this population must be aware of these factors in order to be effective in administrating care. The nurse, being a very important person in the life of the person with AIDS when in the hospital, should provide an atmosphere of individual acceptance of the patient. This means putting aside one's personal feelings or prejudices about the patient's lifestyle or background.[4] Because of the nurse's intimate contact with the patient, the person with AIDS quickly discovers whether the nurse is bringing his or her own agenda to the bedside.[5] The nurse should provide the patient with opportunities to express the strong feelings being experienced during this crucial time.

Anxiety and fear, combined with anger and depression, are often seen in the newly hospitalized AIDS patient. This anxiety may stem partially from not having a specific diagnosis; however, it can also be related to the patient's self-image, since AIDS, like many diseases, can alter one's self-concept.[6]

The terminal stage of AIDS is not well defined. Although life expectancy after diagnosis remains approximately two years, patients have a wide variation in clinical course. Many die during a first acute hospitalization for Pneumocystis carinii pneumonia (PCP).[7] A final phase of irreversible decline is marked by successive, uncontrollable opportunistic infections, progressive general deterioration and debilitation, and often deteriorating mental capacity.[8]

The onset of dementia, successive or multiple opportunistic infections, or irreversible debilitation many signal the need to consider a shift in the focus of treatment from aggressive, active diagnosis and intervention to a palliative approach designed to allow the patient to die in dignity and comfort.[9] AIDS is a miserable disease; those afflicted with it know that they are going to die. Therefore, in discussing cares and concerns, we are talking about where persons with AIDS will receive care, what type of care will be provided, who will provide care, and what the concerns are of those providing care to these terminally ill persons.

Arranging appropriate care for the terminal or chronically and progressively ill AIDS patient can be a challenge. However, in contrast with the typical scenario in a terminal disease such as cancer, multiple opportunistic complications and central nervous system impairment may cause AIDS patients to need intensive, twenty-four-hour personal care and supervision for months before death. The comprehensive approach of hospice care at home is increasingly seen as a model for treatment of patients entering the chronic progressive or terminal stages of AIDS.[10] The goal of hospice care for people with AIDS is to assist the person and family to achieve optimal function and obtain comfort despite the patient's progressive physical and often mental deterioration.[11] But this becomes a special challenge given the unpredictability and severity of the AIDS assault.

Hospice programs, bound to traditional admission criteria of six-month life expectancy, palliative care, and a primary support system, are struggling to admit and care for people with AIDS. Hearing of and experiencing these limitations on admission, people with AIDS often resist being admitted and cared for by hospice programs. By the same token, hospices, traditionally committed to patients whose life expectancy is six months or less, and for whom curative or aggressive therapy has been discontinued, cannot accurately predict life expectancy of AIDS patients at a time when intense research is under way to devise and evaluate new drugs and treatment strategies.[12] One of the critical requirements for working with the person with AIDS is the worker's availability, reliability, empathy, and ability to respond emotionally to the client, particularly during times of regression. The stress placed on the professional by such appropriate expectations cannot be overemphasized.[13]

Dunkel and Hartfield have identified eight countertransference issues associated with the care of the person with AIDS. These include fear of the unknown, fear of contagion, fear of dying and death, denial of helplessness, homophobia, overidentification, anger, and the need to profess omnipotence.[14] As the client nears death, these issues may intensify for the hospice staff. Because of the increasing number of terminally ill AIDS patients, staff can become emotionally overwhelmed with little time to process and reintegrate.[15] One staff member speaks from personal experience:

> AIDS puts a hospice nurse at risk for burnout because there seems to be no predictable course, and the usual methods and treatments that are helpful for cancer patients often do not work for AIDS. In my practice, most of my tried-and-true interventions are not successful. Very little of what I have done or know apply to AIDS except, perhaps, the ability to hang in there until the end—and most of the time I am doing so by only the thinnest thread. The many tricks I have cultivated for hospice patients do not work well with AIDS patients, leaving me feeling frustrated and alone.[16]

Wallace outlines five guidelines that will enable hospice caregivers to cope more effectively with the problems associated with caring for patients with AIDS:

(1) Clarify for AIDS patients and their loved ones what hospice *cannot* do for them before specifying what it *can* do.

(2) Keep your professional footing. Because hospice personnel are usually close in age to AIDS patients and their loved ones, it is easy to overidentify and thus to become enmeshed in patients' struggles to live and die with AIDS.

(3) Learn to listen to your own feelings of helplessness and frustration.

(4) Speak the unspeakable in order to disengage various conflicting values and emotions in the patient family unit.

(5) Get in touch with your own fears about AIDS—fears of contagion, death at a young age, homosexuality, and the drug culture.

Wallace also suggests that by far the most serious and difficult obstacle blocking hospice care for AIDS patients is the lack of primary care persons in the home. Clark et al. have identified AIDS dementia in particular as one of the most difficult complications of this disease to manage at home. Nursing care includes the provision of memory cues; behavioral modification; and the creation of a safe, predictable environment.[17]

WHY HOSPICE?

Changes in reimbursement by health insurance plans are mandating shorter hospital stays. Prospective payments, which originally affected only Medicare patients, are rapidly being expanded to apply to all insurers for all patients. Because of this, hospices have moved into the mainstream of the health care system. The Joint Commission on Accreditation of Hospitals has developed comprehensive standards for the accreditation of hospice programs. Blue Cross/Blue Shield,

Medicare, Medicaid, and most other major third-party payers provide benefits for hospice care.[18] A major rationale for hospice reimbursement by Medicare and other insurance programs is the premise that hospice care, by substituting home care services for hospital inpatient care, is less expensive than conventional care.[19]

In hospice, the unit of care is the entire family, and mandated benefits include the services of physicians, nurses, social workers, and other health professionals in the home, hospital, or nursing home; medication for pain relief and symptom control; medical appliances and equipment; nutrition counseling; extensive health and support services in the home; and bereavement counseling for the patient's family for up to one year.[20] The hospice philosophy seems well suited to care for people with AIDS, especially with the use of a multidisciplinary team. Since no one professional can deal with every issue confronting the patient, the team tends to diffuse the intensity of effort in order not to overwhelm individuals.[21]

The AIDS home care and hospice program, a program of visiting nurses and hospice of San Francisco, uses a multidisciplinary team of nurses, social workers, attendants, and volunteers available on a twenty-four-hour basis in consultation with each patient's primary physician. Some people with AIDS lack any support system. To allow the patient to stay at home, hospice team members may assume this responsibility, including:

- pain and symptom management

- emotional support

- multidisciplinary care team

- pastoral/spiritual counseling

- bereavement counseling

- twenty-four-hour "on-call" nurse/counselor

- staff support.

People with AIDS thus feel secure in the knowledge that there is someone to call on an around-the-clock basis. Remaining at home, while comforting, can be isolating as well: crises often occur at night or on weekends when it is more difficult to contact support systems. Having an on-call nurse to offer advice by telephone or to make a home visit helps to reduce anxiety. Pain may not be as much of a concern for the AIDS patient as diarrhea or difficulty in breathing. The hospice approach emphasizes symptom control and the use of treatments or medications that allow the person to live comfortably.[22]

QUALITY OF CARE

A multidisciplinary team approach entails a comprehensive effort to deal with the patient's medical, social, psychological, and spiritual problems over a period of time and in a variety of settings. These are among the important objectives of a program for the care of the terminal ill. The benefits of a multidisciplinary approach derive from the diversity of talent it brings to the task, but it is most vulnerable in its need for coordination among team members. An important feature of multidisciplinary care in a hospice program is the lack of a sharp distinction between the functions of various team members. Although each has expertise and primary responsibility, each must be alert to the problems and needs of the patient in other areas.[23]

Caring for the person with AIDS or AIDS-Related Complex (ARC) is an unprecedented challenge for those providing home hospice care. Those with AIDS, however, benefit immeasurably from the multidisciplinary approach adopted by most hospice programs; indeed, the physical and psychosocial complexities of AIDS require this sensitive and humane approach.[24] Although many of the home care needs can be met by nurses, the multidisciplinary team, involving social workers, attendants, physical therapists, and volunteers, is essential if the AIDS patient is to remain home. These team members work closely with the primary physician to develop a plan of care that will sustain the person in the home environment. This multidisciplinary approach will help both the patient and the team members deal with the physical and psychological problems related to the diagnosis of AIDS and the terminal stages of the illness, including bereavement support.[25]

Traditional home care does not concern itself that much with bereavement issues. The hospice care program believes in emotional support for the entire family, especially when dealing with death and dying. For the friends and family survivors of an AIDS death, the bereavement process is quite complicated.[26] Skilled bereavement counselors will provide needed support and assistance to the lover, family, and friends of the deceased, even for a period after death has occurred. Zimmerman states that the purpose of hospice bereavement care is to provide comfort, understanding, support, and information to surviving relatives and friends in an effort to alleviate the distress of bereavement and promote the most favorable outcome possible.[27] As members of the hospice team, the social worker and nurse each need to make one or two bereavement follow-up visits; a bereavement volunteer should be assigned to provide ongoing support and counseling to the friends or family members.[28]

HOW TO DEVELOP MORE HOSPICE CARE PROGRAMS FOR PERSONS WITH AIDS

Starting a hospice requires tenacity and adherence to high standards. The obstacles inherent in developing a hospice program, however, loom large, ranging from raising the community's consciousness to the training of staff in the provision of laborious primary nursing care tasks.[29]

Implementation and Coordination

Continuity of care reduces the patient's and the family's sense of alienation and fragmentation; therefore, hospice must be an autonomous and centrally administered program providing a continuum of care to patients and family. Optional utilization of services and sources is an important goal: a governing body (or designated persons) assumes full legal authority and responsibility for the operation of the hospice program. This governing body has written by-laws and oversees administration, services, and fiscal management. A hospice program must maintain written and readily available evidence of its organization, services, and channels of authority.[30]

Hospice programs seek to coordinate their services with professional and nonprofessional services in the community in order to avoid duplication of care. Coordination requires both communication and leadership, and must be evidenced in the organizational structure of each hospice model. Hospice programs must have defined affiliations, linkage, or arrangements for services with one or more facilities, service agencies, or programs along the continuum of care, including acute inpatient care, skilled and intermediate inpatient care, outpatient services, and home care services.[31]

Flexibility and continuity are built into the hospice system of care. Flexibility in the provision of hospice patient care is crucial, due to the frequent changes in the patient's condition and the family's response to the progress of the disease.[32]

And, most important, hospice care is available twenty-four hours a day, seven days a week; since the needs of hospice patients and their families may arise at any time, staff must always be available. Hospice care is intended to be flexible to meet the changing needs of the patient and family. Therefore, a hospice program of care makes its services available to every patient and family on the program, whenever those services are needed. Emphasis is placed on medical and nursing services being available around the clock in the home as well as the inpatient setting.[33]

Dynamic leadership, good staffing, budget flexibility, open communication channels, an active chief executive officer and board interest, democratic involvement in the management decision-making process, and freedom to grow—all assure that the hospice program provides a viable quality service to the community.[34]

PRACTICAL LESSONS FOR STARTING A HOSPICE PROGRAM

Planning

Defined as the making of decisions in the present to bring about an outcome in the future, planning logically precedes all other management functions. Initially, the new hospice group must develop a coherent statement of philosophy or underlying purpose, which provides an overall frame of reference for organizational practice; it lays the foundation of goals, objectives, policies, and derived plans.[35] Currently, a "mission statement" is required as an overall goal for the hospice organization. A standard mission statement should read as follows when the focus is on the care of persons with AIDS:

Hospice, a community-based model of care, is a program of palliative and supportive services which provides physical, psychological, social, and spiritual care for terminally ill persons with AIDS and their families. Services are provided by a medically supervised multi-disciplinary team of professionals and volunteers. Hospice services are available in both home and an inpatient setting: home care is provided on a part-time, intermittent, regularly scheduled, and around-the-clock basis. Bereavement services are available to the family. Admission to a hospice program of care is on the basis of patient and family need. Hospice provides a comprehensive continuation of care utilizing an integration of appropriate services to eliminate duplication and fragmentation. Hospice affirms life. Hospice exists to provide support and care for persons in the last phases of incurable illness. Hospice recognizes dying as a normal process, whether or not resulting from disease. Hospice neither hastens nor postpones death. Hospice exists in the hopes and belief that, through appropriate care and the promotion of a caring community sensitive to their needs, patients and families may be free to attain a degree of mental and spiritual preparation for death that is satisfactory to them.

Hospice is a community-based program of specialized health care which does not end when acute care is completed. Total patient care extends even beyond, to his surviving family. Hospice teaches a new attitude toward dying and death as the realization and conscious acceptance of dying and death as part of being born and part of the struggle of life. The concept of hospice is that the terminally ill person with AIDS should be allowed to die at home or in surroundings more home-like and congenial than the usual hospice setting.[36]

Developing a Viable Organizational Structure

All organizations have a structure, which is frequently written out as an organizational chart.[37] The organizational chart for hospice programs will vary according to the model of care. When developing a hospice care center for persons with AIDS, be sure to specify types and location of services.

Forming Committees

The committee is paramount to the organizational process. Once the board of directors is appointed, the key committees must be selected from a cross section of the community.[38] This is a very important consideration when developing hospice care programs for persons with AIDS; if the community is against the center being developed in their neighborhood, they will protest against it. The commitment to a cause or program by neighborhood leaders and workers often leads to future success. As leaders in a locally based organization, hospice administrators cannot ignore the potential impact of community support.[39] This support not only promotes funding and patronage, but also determines volunteer contributions and staffing patterns. Liaisons with churches, civic organizations, and related groups help promote the concept of hospice care and encourage the contribution of available resources.[40]

In the organization and administration of hospice, active committees are valuable to the manager as a mechanism for progress. Committee activities allow directors of hospice programs more time to spend in managing care. McDonnell feels that, initially, committee membership should include those who were involved in the formulation of objectives for psychiatrists, clergy, bereavement counselors, nurses, social workers, and therapists.[41]

Developing Programs

Program adoption requires the cooperation of those involved in developing objectives and investigating external influences such as environmental problems and constraints. Programs design furnishes a base for development of polices that reflect the hospice model.[42]

When developing programs for hospice care programs it is essential to remember that AIDS patients' needs are different from those of traditional hospice care patients. Significantly, they risk contracting an opportunistic infection at any time. Program components requiring development for any viable hospice program of care include:

- education
- volunteer services
- home care
- inpatient care
- bereavement support
- outpatient care

Effective Staffing

A smooth program is marked by teamwork and team spirit. Staff members need mutual support.[43] Volunteers are as important as professionals; they will be needed in increasing numbers as more community-based facilities are developed as alternatives to hospitalization for persons with AIDS.[44] A beginning community hospice group will generally include nurses, secretaries, social workers, attorneys, and laypeople who have worked through personal loss. These people supply a wealth of talent and experience on which to build a successful hospice program.[45]

What is needed in all hospice programs is a group of hardy people able to stand up to the pressures of a medical staff who is likely to be less than enthusiastic—people who are more motivated by challenge, responsibility, autonomy, and recognition than by financial or job security.[46] Recruiting staff and volunteer caregivers for people with AIDS requires health professionals to deal directly with the complex issues that AIDS has introduced into our society.

These are some of the issues which volunteer caretakers must face before they can be effective and cope personally with the stresses implicit in their role.[47]

Staff selection and staffing patterns provide a key element in the implementation of a successful program. Hasty selection may result in the recruitment of professionals who lack a basic understanding of the hospice concept.[48]

Seeking Funding Sources

Most hospice models have utilized the traditional reimbursement sources for revenues in order to provide an ongoing funding mechanism. For beginning hospice programs, third-party reimbursement is a critical factor. While grant awards are welcomed for program development, they should not be the only beginning source of income.[49]

Hospice is now being viewed by business coalitions, industry, health professionals, and hospital administrators as an alternative delivery system, alongside health maintenance and preferred provider organizations. Business, labor, and provider leaders have recognized the importance of containing health care costs; alternative health delivery systems increase competition and introduce marketplace incentives to keep the costs of health care down. The advantages of hospice must be explored on the basis of cost as well as quality, access to care, benefits, and delivery system characteristics.[50]

Establishing a Referral Source

Unless hospice administrators establish appropriate linkage with community agencies and various facilities in the community to bring the hospice program closer to existing and future patients, referrals will be limited, with other providers coming forth as competitors rather than as supporters.[51]

Establishing a referral source for a hospice that will deal primarily with persons with AIDS is very important. According to Richard Ames: "What will be a hospice program's primary area of service? It will be partially defined by whether a hospice is community- or institution-based and by the hospice's source of referrals. What geographic or population area will it cover? . . . I suggest starting with the obvious. Begin with whatever population obviously needs care."[52]

Community agencies that sponsor educational programs make good referral sources. McDonnell states that word-of-mouth provides an important source for referrals, and is enhanced by the provision of good services.[53] If referral sources are not secure, the hospice program may not survive.

Initiating Public Relations

A communication and education network established early in the planning stage provides a base for hospice acceptance. This is a very important step in educating the public about AIDS and its modes of transmission. Traditional media sources—newspapers, radio, and television—can tell the story very effectively in interviews and features about services provided to people with AIDS. Public service announcements, articles about hospice programs for AIDS patients, and panel discussions are only a few of the many approaches possible.

Nurturing Community Support

With hospice being in constant interaction with the environment, it is highly important to reckon with the appropriate forces in the community. The inclusion of a large number of people within the community in the various hospice committees allows both input and a way of marketing. Hospice appointments to board committees must include health and other professionals—lawyers, realtors, engineers, bankers, accountants, and representatives from educational institutions, church groups, service clubs, auxiliaries, business, labor, industry, and the media—providing a real cross section of the community.[54]

Evaluation and Research

A major responsibility of hospice program administrators is the attainment of desired goals and objectives in a cost-effective manner. Evaluation of hospice program components must be carried out on an annual basis or more often if necessary.[55]

McDonnell states that one community-based model carries out an evaluation of its program by having each patient complete a form. The survey is designed for families who have participated in the program and is used to promote quality care. Another hospice has a program evaluation format to meet function requirements involving board and committee review of administration, services, staffing, and finance.[56]

Accreditation by the Joint Commission on Accreditation of Health Care Organizations (JCAHO) provides both a self-evaluation mechanism and a tool for research. The Medicare hospice regulation requires that all participating hospice organizations file cost reports with the Health Care Financing Administration (HCFA). The accumulation of such cost statistics will provide the widest body of information yet assembled on hospice characteristics, utilization, and costs; the resulting data base will be helpful in further research. Because of mandated data collection and analysis, we will be able to assess objectively the true values of hospices.[57]

Hospice care is an excellent setting for research projects because it blends existing disciplines to achieve one goal in order that care may be administered holistically. Limited studies have been done on the effects of counseling the dying and their families, the outcomes of a bereavement program, the approaches to care for the chronically ill and elderly, the use of volunteers in health care, the family and patient as a "single unit of care," and the numerous other aspects of care which hospice brings, for the first time, to the health care system. Since hospice may be a real agent for change in the American health care delivery system, hospice managers must be alert to its extremely important role in future research. Added research into satisfaction indexes of patients, families, and professionals is also vital to hospice programs.[58]

THE ETHICS OF HOSPICE CARE

The ethics of hospice care has to do with how caregivers make choices in the case of the terminally ill. Such caregivers are confronted with questions of what they ought to be and what is right or good for their patients.[59]

Ethics is concerned not only with choices but with the values through which choices are given their importance and persuasiveness. The ethics of hospice care includes not only what caregivers do, but why they do what they do. Obviously, bringing the values of hospice care into focus does not eliminate all moral problems in the care of the terminally ill. Davidson states that such a discussion nevertheless should provide greater opportunity to make choices consistent with values as care is rendered.[60]

The notion of hospice resists simple definitions, partly because it is itself a moral notion. As a team, hospice is impossible to define without addressing the issues of the quality of life and how people ought to die. It should be emphasized that hospice is not primarily a place, but a concept of care which can be actualized to a greater or lesser degree in a variety of settings.[61]

CONCLUSION

Many concerns and complications surround the development of more hospice center programs for persons with AIDS. One particular complication is a community's resistance to a hospice center being built in their neighborhood, especially if its target population will be AIDS patients. A tangential concern of this chapter has been the fear and stigma surrounding AIDS. Therefore, getting a community to agree to develop a hospice in their neighborhood will take a lot of work and persuasion.

Starting a hospice for persons with AIDS requires tenacity, high standards, and a combination of inpatient and home care services. It must be clearly defined how AIDS patients will be served. But, because the goal of hospice care is to assist the dying and their families to achieve optimal function and comfort, hospice centers provide the best alternative for the care of people with AIDS. Furthermore, with the number of AIDS-related deaths steadily rising, there will be a push for cost containment and endorsement of certain types of health care. By participating in health and community planning, hospices can be at the forefront in offering care to people with AIDS.

Ability and know-how in the development of more hospice centers are steadily on the rise. In implementing their goals, hospice caregivers to people with AIDS should keep an ever open mind to the special needs and concerns of those afflicted with this dreadful disease.

NOTES

1. Jerry D. Durham and Felissa L. Cohen, *The Person with AIDS* (New York: Springer Publishing Company, 1987), pp. 21–37.
2. Ibid.
3. Ibid.
4. Ibid.
5. Ibid.
6. Ibid.
7. D. I. Abrams et al., "AIDS: Caring for the Dying Patient," *Patient Care* 23, no. 19 (November 30, 1989).
8. Ibid., p. 26.
9. Ibid., pp. 29–32.
10. Ibid., pp. 34–36
11. C. Clark et al., "Hospice Care: A Model for Caring for the Person with AIDS," *Nursing Clinics of North America* 23 (1988): 851–62.
12. Abrams et al., "AIDS: Caring for the Dying Patient," p. 23.
13. Clark et al., "Hospice Care," pp. 851–62.
14. Ibid.
15. Ibid.
16. T. Stephany "AIDS and the Hospice Nurse," *Home Health Nurse* 8, no. 2 (March–April 1990): 141–54.
17. Clark et al., "Hospice Care," pp. 851–62.
18. W. Bulkin, and H. Lukashok, "Rx for Dying: The Case for Hospice," *New England Journal of Medicine* 318, no. 6 (February 11, 1988): 316–18.
19. J. Rhymes "Hospice Care in America," *Journal of the American Medical Association* 264, no. 3 (July 18, 1990): 369–72.
20. Bulkin and Lukashok, "Rx for Dying: The Case for Hospice."
21. Clark et al., "Hospice Care," pp. 851–62.
22. Ibid.

23. Jack McKay Zimmerman, *Hospice: Complete Care for the Terminally Ill* (Baltimore–Munich: Urban and Schwarzenberg, 1986), pp. 98–112.

24. Inge B. Corless and Mory Pittman-Lindeman, *AIDS Principles, Practice, and Politics* (New York: Hemisphere Publishing Corporation, 1989), pp. 58–72.

25. Durham and Cohen, *The Person with AIDS*, pp. 21–37.

26. Clark et al., "Hospice Care," pp. 851–62.

27. Zimmerman, *Hospice: Complete Care for the Terminally Ill*, pp. 98–112.

28. Durham and Cohen, *The Person with AIDS*, pp. 21–37.

29. Richard P. Ames, "Starting a Hospice Requires Tenacity, High Standards," *Hospital Progress* 61 (1989): 56–59.

30. Alice McDonnell, *Quality Hospice Care: Administration, Organization, and Models* (Owings Mills, Md.: National Health Publishing, 1986), pp. 141–62.

31. Ibid.

32. Ibid.

33. Ibid.

34. Ibid.

35. Ibid.

36. Ibid.

37. Ibid.

38. Ibid.

39. Lenora Paradis, *Hospice Handbook: A Guide for Managers and Planners* (Rockville, Md.: Aspen Publications, Inc., 1985), pp. 81–111.

40. Ibid.

41. McDonnell, *Quality Hospice Care*, pp. 141–62.

42. Ibid.

43. Ames, "Starting a Hospice Program Requires Tenacity, High Standards," pp 56–59.

44. M. A. Jimenez and D. R. Jimenez, "Training Volunteer Caregivers of Persons with AIDS," *Social Work Health Care* 14, no. 3 (1990): 73–85.

45. Ames, "Starting a Hospice Program Requires Tenacity, High Standards," pp 56–59.

46. McDonnell, *Quality Hospice Care.*

47. Jimenez and Jimenez, "Training Volunteer Caregivers of Persons with AIDS."

48. McDonnell, *Quality Hospice Care.*

49. Ibid.

50. Ibid.

51. Ibid.

52. Ames, "Starting a Hospice Program Requires Tenacity, High Standards," pp 56–59.

53. McDonnell, *Quality Hospice Care.*

54. Ibid.

55. Ibid.

56. Ibid.

57. Ibid.

58. Ibid.

59. Glen W. Davidson, *The Hospice: Development and Administration,* 2d ed. (Washington, D.C.: Hemisphere Publishing Corporation, 1985), pp. 149–66.

60. Ibid.

61. Ibid.

6

Hospice Care for Children with AIDS
(with Connie Wolf)

Adults are not the only group affected by AIDS. The World Health Organization (WHO) projects that by the year 2000, HIV infections in men, women, and children will total about 40 million. Of this cumulative total, WHO estimates that 10 million infants and children worldwide will have been infected with the virus, with the majority dying of AIDS. An equally disturbing projection is that by the end of this decade, more than 10 million children will be orphaned due to one or both parents dying of AIDS.[1]

In the decade since the epidemic began, an estimated 400,000 cases of AIDS have occurred among infants and children under five years of age, with 90 percent of these cases occurring in sub-Saharan Africa.[2] In the United States, 2,789 cases of AIDS in children under thirteen years of age were reported to the Centers for Disease Control (CDC) as of December 1990. More than half of these children have already died. Eighty-four percent of these cases were due to perinatal infection. In addition, the rate of increase has risen 37 percent from 1987.[3] Through the past thirty years, the contributions of cancer and other major causes of death in children have remained stable. However, the effect of HIV infection is rapidly increasing. Already among the ten leading causes of death in infants, young children, and adolescents, AIDS will probably move into the top five causes within the next several years.[4]

The increasing rates of HIV infection in the United States, as well as in other nations around the world, are startling. Now, because of the significantly higher number of cases of children with AIDS, health care providers will be facing an even greater challenge. In the final stages of the disease, hospice care can be beneficial for children and their families, just as it can be for adults with AIDS. To comprehend and deal effectively with the issue of children with AIDS, several points need to be considered. This chapter will discuss the transmission and detection of HIV infection in children along with the psychosocial impacts of the disease. Then, focus will turn to foster care and to the options presented by hospice care during the final stages of AIDS in the dying child. Finally, specific hospice programs will be discussed.

TRANSMISSION OF HIV IN CHILDREN

Transmission of HIV in children usually occurs through one of three routes: perinatal infection, transfusion of contaminated blood, or sexual exposure. Perinatal infection is the most common and involves vertical transmission of the virus from mother to child either across the placenta or during birth. Almost 79 percent of women with AIDS are in their child-bearing years. In the United States and Europe, most cases of perinatal transmission were observed in women who were intravenous (IV)-drug users themselves (52 percent), or who had had sexual intercourse with a partner who was an IV-drug user (21 percent). Most women who gave birth to an HIV-infected infant showed no symptoms themselves at delivery. Also, not every child born to an HIV-infected mother will be infected. Current studies suggest that transmission occurs in about one-third of infants born to HIV-infected mothers. Although not yet clearly defined. certain factors may influence transmission; these include the severity of maternal infection, extent of viremia (virus in the bloodstream) and growth of the infection, genetic factors, and other cofactors.[5] Among pregnant women or newborn infants, HIV disproportionately affects minorities: blacks constitute 53 percent of AIDS cases in children, and Hispanics 23 percent.[6]

As far as other modes of transmission, a small number of cases have been reported in which the infant was infected with HIV postpartum through breast feeding. Also, some children were infected through contaminated transfusions before 1985, when the nationwide screening procedures were instituted. In extremely rare cases, children became infected through sexual abuse.[7]

Transmission of HIV among adolescents occurs primarily through sexual contact (heterosexual and homosexual) with infected persons; infection from contaminated blood and blood products and intravenous drug use have also been reported.[8] The U.S. Department of Education has estimated that by age fifteen, 16 percent of males and 5 percent of females have had sexual intercourse at least once. The numbers rapidly increase in the later teens: by age nineteen, figures rise to 75 percent for males and 67 percent for females.[9] Even though these young people may know how AIDS is transmitted, most of them are not using condoms, which would provide some protection against transmission. Risk of contracting HIV increases as a result of widespread drug abuse among teenagers. In a recent study, it was found that 20,000 teens reported using drugs intravenously at least once.[10] The activities of adolescent runaways and teenage prostitutes place this group as a whole at an even greater risk.[11]

DETECTION OF HIV IN CHILDREN

In children, it is often difficult to describe and detect AIDS because the disease must be differentiated from other congenital and immunodeficiency diseases.[12] Signs and symptoms of AIDS in children include failure to grow and develop, and recurrent bacterial infections. These infections may be inner ear infections, chronic inflammation of the lungs, thrush, and/or swollen lymph nodes.[13] With chronic inflammations and infections, eating may become difficult, thus making adequate nutrition hard to attain. Due to this, children may experience subsequent weight loss, chronic diarrhea, shortness of breath, fatigue, and impaired growth.

Neurological effects may involve cognitive impairment, regression in development, and/or delay in achievement of certain developmental milestones. For example, children may stop feeding themselves or resort to crawling instead of walking.[14] Children with AIDS may also show other symptoms such as dizziness, fever and night sweats, swollen glands, heavy cough, purple or discolored growths on the skin, and/or unexplained bleeding from any body opening.[15]

THE PSYCHOSOCIAL IMPACT OF AIDS ON CHILDREN AND THEIR FAMILIES

AIDS has not only physical consequences but psychosocial ones as well. Certain psychological symptoms may accompany brain infections that result from the loss of normal immune functions. Other psychological symptoms may be related to the child's own fear of death or to other people's reactions to the child's illness.[16]

Often children with AIDS blame themselves for their disease. They may see pain as their punishment and attribute the illness to recent family interactions.[17] They may feel guilty and experience sadness, hopelessness, helplessness, isolation, and depression. Some may think about suicide as they realize that AIDS will eventually progress to pain and death.[18]

With increased hospitalization, children with AIDS may face pain, separation from family and home, and medical routines and procedures that may hurt and/or scare them. They may also experience the isolation that can result from the actions of hospital staff, family members, and visitors. The often fearful behaviors of these people will be felt by the ill child. Such actions may inhibit the intimate touching that a child needs for normal development. Therefore, these children, in their uncertain and isolated environment, will not experience the security and love that unaffected children do.[19] To combat the isolation, children may acquire a lowered sense of self-worth or maladaptive defenses, including loss of affect, pathological denial, depression, and possibly greater developmental disturbances. For the child with AIDS, the most traumatic aspect of the illness is probably separation.[20] Dr. Belfer, professor and chairman of the Child Psychiatry Department of Harvard Medical School at Cambridge Hospital, reports, "These children and adolescents are modern lepers. This is a new and horrifying psychological burden for the child."[21]

When a family member is infected with HIV, uncertainty and stress overwhelm the family as a whole. Many fears surface, such as loss of confidentiality; stigmatization; isolation; abandonment by family, friends, neighbors, and co-workers; loss of housing; and loss of employment. These fears call for support and counseling from psychologists, social workers, or other mental health professionals. Many times affected families are of lower socioeconomic status, and AIDS further inhibits their efforts to be self-sufficient. Since they may not be able to afford medical insurance, special needs arise for financial assistance and social services.[22]

All aspects of family life (social roles, economic functioning, and relationships) are affected by the illness of a family member. Apart from accepting the diagnosis of AIDS, the family may have to deal with issues such as drug use, homosexuality, and/or prostitution if they play a role in the situation. Parents of a child with AIDS may feel the pain of separation due to hospitalization of their child. Further complications arise for the mother who has passed HIV onto her child, because she must also come to terms with her own illness. She may feel overwhelming guilt, especially if she is not yet ill herself. Finally, families affected by AIDS may experience public condemnation and fear. This often results in withdrawal of social support at a time when it is most needed.[23,24,25]

Because of the proliferation of AIDS among the young, even children who are not HIV-infected often show incredible fear of contracting AIDS themselves. As a result, they are at a higher risk for anorexia, apathy, and social withdrawal.[26] The following case studies are illustrative.

Case Study

A thirteen-year-old boy, preoccupied with fears of contracting and transmitting AIDS, was shown to have a six-week history of cleaning and checking rituals. These thoughts were closely linked to his intense handwashing and associated with avoidant behavior. For instance, he did not watch television for fear that AIDS or homosexuality would be mentioned or intimate physical contact portrayed.

The acute onset of symptoms followed a school biology lesson devoted to "germs" and coincided with the government-sponsored AIDS campaign that saturated the media. Soon afterward, the boy's life was severely limited, with two-thirds of each day spent in ritualized activity. He had completely withdrawn from school and other social contact, and was unable to venture from his home.

The patient, the elder of two children of an intact family, had no previous psychiatric history, nor did anyone else in his family. There was no history of sexual abuse or experimentation, and indeed, his psychosexual development lagged behind that of his peers. He was an unassertive, meticulous boy, who had always lacked confidence and showed anxiety in novel situations. He also poorly identified with his father, who was peripheral within the family.

A response prevention program, with both individual and family support, helped him to return to school and abandon many of his rituals. His central fear of AIDS and some of the attendant avoidant behavior, however, are still prominent.[27]

Case Study

A twelve-year-old boy, the eldest of four children from an intact family, was referred with serious emotional and behavioral problems. He was reported as disruptive, having poor concentration, an under-achiever by his school, and difficult to manage by his family.

The major problem prompting referral was that he had become particularly upset shortly after going to bed in the past several months. He had developed the habit of coming downstairs in tears to seek comfort each evening. He had recently revealed to his parents that this habit was related to extreme fear that he would contract AIDS.

This young man presented as physically mature for his age. He talked with evident emotion about AIDS at a second interview, saying that he felt ignorant about it, and as a result, believed it was inevitable that he would catch AIDS. Here he clearly referred to the television publicity material and particularly to the statement, "Don't Die of Ignorance." It was clear that this material had precipitated his distress.

There are many likely causes of this boy's problems. Temperamental features and a possible early anxious attachment were felt to be important background aspects. His conduct difficulties also probably reflected underachievement due to a mild hearing loss still under treatment and family structural problems.

At the next interview, both the patient and his family reported a major improvement in both his emotional upset and behavior since the previous discussion. Happily, this improvement was progressive and sustained.[28]

With this lack of education among children comes a common prejudice against people with AIDS. Little is known about the knowledge and attitudes that normal children have about AIDS. A study of 908 seventh- and tenth-grade students in two school districts in Rhode Island showed that 55 percent of the students would not chance touching a student with AIDS and that 38 percent felt AIDS patients should not be allowed in school. However, 90 percent of the children knew that casual contact could not transmit the disease. Also, 45 percent of them felt that homosexuals were the sole cause of the AIDS crisis.[29] These results reiterate the need for increased education on this issue.

FOSTER CARE FOR THE CHILD WITH AIDS

Additional care beyond the extended family is sometimes necessary for families with HIV. Due to its relationship to intravenous drug abuse, pediatric HIV infection is most often a disease of poverty. A family may be disabled by drug abuse to the point where care even for a healthy child would be difficult, and impossible for an HIV-infected child. Therefore, foster care may be necessary in these situations.

Numerous problems exist in recruiting foster families for HIV-infected children. Since the infected child will suffer physical and psychological problems, the foster parents must be prepared to handle these situations as they arise. Not many people are willing to take on this type of responsibility. Potential foster families are intimidated, and few are willing to deal with the burden of the HIV-infected child. Although the number of children with AIDS is increasing, the number of people willing to care for them remains small.

New measures are being taken to increase the pool of foster parents. Financial incentives are being offered; also, nontraditional candidates (e.g., single men and gay couples) are being approved. For families who take in more than one infected child, home health aides and homemakers are provided. Still, there are not enough foster families to meet the number of children who need to be placed.

Prior to placement in a foster family, a child may enter a transitional care facility. St. Clare's Home for Children in Virginia is one example. St. Clare's is run with the philosophy that "children belong within the family structure and the ultimate goal is placement in a loving and stable home." Presently, these transitional group homes operate on a small scale. However, they are effective and may be utilized more in the future.

HOSPICE CARE FOR THE CHILD WITH AIDS

Children with AIDS and their families need a special kind of care adapted to their many needs. Tertiary care is required for the management of the acute medical problems faced by the AIDS patient and for the minimization of exposure of the immunosuppressed child to infectious agents. The child and family also require social support to meet their psychosocial needs. Because of these varied requirements, hospice care is well suited for children with AIDS and their families.

The admission to a children's hospice program is made on the basis of the patient's and family's needs. Whereas many health care providers base admission on need for services as well as on the ability to pay, hospice emphasizes true care for the dying child and mourning family.[30] This reflects the idealistic and noninstitutional foundation of the hospice movement.

When hospice care first began, terminally ill cancer patients were the initial referrals. Today, there is no diagnostic requirement in hospice care. In 1986, over 9,000 people died from AIDS; hospice care served 23 percent of these people. The number of patients served by hospice care has since doubled.[31] Hospice provides an ideal environment not just for the cancer patient but for the terminally ill AIDS patient as well. People need to be told that hospice may be an available alternative to them.

Children's Hospice International (CHI) is a well-known program in the United States, which is most noted for the CHI "circle of care." Medicine, nursing, psychology, social service, spiritual support, support groups, therapists, volunteers, academic institutions, community relations, home care, and hospitals are all aspects of this "circle of care."[32] CHI has promoted four interrelated goals: the hospice philosophy throughout pediatric facilities, inclusion of children in existing hospice programs, inclusion of the hospice perspective in existing hospice programs, and increasing the public's awareness of terminally ill children's needs.[33]

Hospice care programs focus on keeping the patient pain-free and as comfortable as possible. Hospice workers assist dying patients and their families so that the patients can live their final days to the fullest and with dignity. Because of the intensity of any terminal illness, the team approach is used in hospice care; no one professional could deal alone with the many different issues that patients and families may face. The team can provide pain and symptom management, emotional support, spiritual counseling, bereavement counseling, twenty-four-hour "on-call" services, and general staff support. All the members of the hospice team, consisting of the pediatrician, primary nurse, social worker, psychologist, trained volunteers, therapists, and clergy,[34] focus on the physical, psychosocial, and spiritual needs of each child and family.

The roles of all team members are important. The pediatrician has many responsibilities, including prescribing pain medication and ordering diagnostic studies when needed. The primary nurse assesses the child's physical condition, provides interventions, and discusses changes in the child's condition with the pediatrician.

The major units of attention for the social worker include the child, the family, the staff, and the service network. The transactions that occur between the child and his or her environment become very important as the social worker aids in the young person's adjustment to the hospice program. The social worker is also concerned with the child's ability to cope with routine daily tasks related to the different stages of the disease. Programs may be set up to deal with problem-solving activities, painful and hurtful emotions, the child's sense of self-worth, and decision making. The social worker must anticipate changes in the child's outlook as well as changes in the disease as it progresses.[35]

The psychologist on the hospice team can play a central role in any effort pertaining to the family's medical and psychosocial concerns by serving as a link between the family and the pediatrician. Psychologists can also provide case consultation to the other team members on the social and emotional issues affecting child and family in relation to the disease. Because HIV may affect the child's central nervous system, thus producing psychological symptoms, the psychologist can aid in evaluating the degree and extent of the complications, and can also help with decisions regarding the types of educational and therapeutic interventions that the child may require.[36]

Another important member of any hospice team is the volunteer. Volunteers work with all members of the team. They may take the burden off the professional staff, replenishing their enthusiasm and preventing staff "burnout." They may also work closely with the child and family. The volunteer can form a tight relationship with a dying child, something the others may not be able to do. For example, the pediatrician may be seen as the bearer of bad news because he or she "pokes needles" into the child. The bond that can form between the dying child and the volunteer is extremely important, since the child may be feeling vulnerable, scared, and lonely. Volunteers go through an intense training process in which they learn strategies to work effectively with the child, the family, and other members of the hospice team during these tough times. They may also assist in several other areas, including transportation, massage therapy, spiritual support, and bereavement.[37]

A physical or rehabilitational therapist may serve as part of the hospice team. Maximizing the child's movement and helping the youngster use resources most efficiently are some of the therapist's goals.

Because the dying child may have spiritual questions, clergy play a role on the hospice team. Even if the child is too young to understand clearly what is happening, the family may have concerns and questions that can be discussed with clergy. During a terminal illness, the outward personality of a patient is often stripped away, revealing the person's inner self. As one dying boy told his mother, "My real self is coming out with this illness."

In hospice, the integration of all contributors of care into one team is essential—this includes the dying child and his or her family. The patient is in fact the most important member of the team. The child, along with the family if possible, decides on the treatment and the type and amount of social interactions. Unfortunately, some children have parents who are no longer living; some are alienated from their families; and some were brought up in uncaring environments. If the child with AIDS does not have a supportive family, a support team is provided.

The assurance of a "safe passageway" for the dying child and family is necessary. This involves the continuum of care right up to the death of the child. Services are also provided for the family after the child's death.[38] All team members take part in attaining this high level of care.

It is left up to the child and family to decide which hospice model to employ. Home care for the HIV-infected child may be quite appropriate; in situations where children are infected with the virus but are not yet showing acute symptoms, they should be allowed to continue to live a normal childhood. However, problems may arise since AIDS arouses fear in many people, who still do not understand the routes of transmission of HIV and wrongly believe that it can be transmitted through casual contact. People also stereotype the lifestyles of HIV-infected patients. Parents of infected children and the health care providers who serve them should be made aware of the possibility of the condition being known in the educational setting and the problems that may develop because of this. The hospice team must be prepared to talk openly with children about such problems. This outlet is extremely important in preventing a child's frustrations from compounding.

If the family does decide on home care for the HIV-infected child, a few precautions should be followed. To prevent acquisition of HIV during home care of infected patients, the Medical Society of New York has issued the following guidelines:

HIV-infected persons can be safely cared for in home environments. In studies of HIV-infected persons and their families, no evidence of transmission of HIV to adults who were not sexual contacts or to children who were not at risk for perinatal transmission was found. Risk of transmission of infection to health care workers in the home setting is the same as the risk for health care workers in other health settings.

In the home setting, it is appropriate to use measures similar to those used in a hospital setting. Needles should not be recapped, purposefully bent, broken, removed from disposable syringes, or otherwise manipulated by hand. Puncture-resistant containers should be used for disposal of needles and other sharp items. Local regulations should be followed for disposal of solid waste. Blood and other body fluids should be flushed down the toilet. Contaminated items that cannot be flushed down the toilet would be wrapped securely in a plastic bag that is sturdy and not easily penetrated. The plastic bag should be placed in a second bag and then should be discarded in a manner consistent with local regulations. Soap and water or other household detergents should be used to clean up spills of blood and other body fluids. Disposable gloves should be worn when cleaning up these spills. After cleaning the exposed area, a disinfectant solution or a freshly prepared solution of sodium hypochlorite (household bleach) should be administered.[39]

Understanding a child's concept of death is pertinent to the care provided by the hospice team. In infants, there is difficulty in the intellectual understanding of the meaning of death; however, infants do have a sense of separation, especially from their mothers.[40] The infant's sense of loss can be seen in a variety of symptoms: easy irritability, crying, weight loss, and apathy are a few.[41] The hospice team should encourage family visits and allow the family to hold the baby. Because the HIV-infected baby may be quiet and withdrawn—characteristics that may be viewed mistakenly as traits of a "good baby"—the hospice staff should be encouraged to hold, play with, and talk to the baby. These babies need the same loving and caring attention that uninfected babies would receive.[42]

The toddler's concept of death remains limited as well, but small ideas of "being" and "nonbeing" are developing at this age. Parents should interact with hospice staff in the child's presence; therefore, the child will begin to trust the staff. The child should be allowed to vent anger and feelings of anxiety, and then be redirected to playing and learning activities. To make up for possible sibling loss, the child should be encouraged to interact with other children. Also, superficial attachment to staff should be discouraged, and caring should be steady. If the family is unable to give consistent care, family services will be provided.[43]

Beyond the toddler stage, the child's view of death may vary quite extensively. At this age, communication becomes increasingly important. Communicating with a dying child in his or her final stage of life is a delicate process that requires a clear understanding of the goals and purposes of such interactions. To help reduce anxiety and fear, telling the child factual information about death may be helpful. Communication is the child's link to emotional support. Talking with a dying child can range from routine discussion to a deep, intensely personal, spiritual experience.

Answering the following questions may help clarify communication with a dying child:

(1) Is there a specific agenda in mind, such as reducing depression, increasing medical compliance, or exploring spirituality; or is the communication nonspecific and supportive?

(2) What are the expectations for accomplishment which the child, parents, and/or hospice workers associate with the communication? Are the goals consistent within the team?

(3) What is the level of comfort of the person talking with the dying child?

The content of the discussion with the dying child needs to be based on the following characteristics: age; level of understanding; sex; family network and support staff; values of the child, including religion and ethnic ideas about death and dying; medical experiences; coping strategies; pain management; the child's ability to respond to detail; and current health status.

Rapport with the children is the first thing that must be established. Cues must be taken from the children in order to question their concerns in a way that meets their needs. The decisions that any child may make must be respected. Useful strategies for talking include one-on-one conversation; consistency in being with the children on a continual basis; play therapy or joining the children in their games; and metaphorical communication, which involves the ability to present ideas to the children in nonthreatening ways. Using fairy tales to make a point is a good example of metaphorical communication.[44]

At birth a child begins using physical, social, and environmental interactions. Play is an important tool when relating to the HIV-infected child; it helps a child develop adaptive skills such as discovering opportunities and being competent in exploration of the environment. A child's self-concept can often be seen through play activity. Many times HIV-infected children display withdrawal, anxiety, or non-communicative behaviors. Creative activities and discovery of new interests are critical components in raising the child's self-esteem.[45]

Through artwork children are able to communicate their real feelings; artwork provides a somewhat nonthreatening way for children to discuss fears of dying and possible prejudices and hurts that they may experience with AIDS. To interpret a child's drawings, it is important to recognize that a child's unconscious can express itself in spontaneous ways, that drawings are a real and original means of communication, and that a child's body and psyche are interlinked and this bonding allows for continuous communication between the two. Interpretation of artwork involves looking for objects that may be present or missing in the drawings. This may symbolize something. Asking about feelings or ideas the child has on each object is important, as well as understanding the real reflection of the picture. The most crucial element in understanding dying children is the ability to be sensitive and caring to their feelings and actions.[46]

Case Study

"Robbie's" death was unexpected and everyone involved was shocked: his family, the nurses, the physicians, and his young roommate, Jimmy. Initially, Jimmy's mother insisted that he not be informed of Robbie's death. Instead, she would tell Jimmy that his new-found friend had been transferred to another ward. After much encouragement from the nursing staff, she finally relented to share the truth with Jimmy. However, she requested that one of the nurses tell her son about Robbie's death because of her own discomfort and anxiety.

After explaining to Jimmy the factors contributing to Robbie's death, in a manner that the youngster could comprehend, the nurse ended the account by saying, "Robbie died and is in heaven now." Jimmy immediately interjected with, "No, he's not! He can't be." "What do you mean?" the nurse asked, obviously concealing her unnerved feeling in response to his brash disclaimer. "Well," Jimmy began slowly, "Robbie couldn't be in heaven already; it took the astronauts three days to get to the moon; it'll take Robbie a lot longer to get to heaven!"[47]

This case study illustrates that a child's concept of death differs greatly from that of adults and is further differentiated by age groups and maturity.[48] Hospice care workers can help the child and family explore thoughts on dying and other related issues.

Dying children experience pain and grief, and their siblings may face similar feelings, too. Physical illness, withdrawal, guilt, and insomnia are all conditions a sibling may experience when a brother or sister dies from AIDS. Hospice care provides an art therapy for bereaved youth; this idea was developed by the Grand Traverse Area Hospice of Munson Medical Center in 1985. The goals of this group were to help clarify the child's feelings about death, to help him or her understand that others feel the same way, to give the sibling the opportunity to learn communication and coping skills, and to give him or her the chance to explore future attitudes about love relationships. Group activities include music, movement, and art; all aid in the sibling's development of new ways of expression. Other exercises include trust walks, goodbye and hello dances, and breathing strategies. Through these exercises, a sibling can rebuild trust after the loss of a loved one, learn ways to accept feelings, and develop a sense of control.[49]

HOSPICE PROGRAMS FOR CHILDREN WITH AIDS

Numerous programs in the United States provide care for HIV-infected children. This section contains brief descriptions of some of these programs.

The Dallas-Fort Worth Area Pediatric AIDS Health Care Demonstration is located at the University of Texas. The project's goals include providing family-oriented model programs; serving medical, psychological, developmental, educational, and basic human rights; and assisting with family unity and support needs of HIV-infected infants, children, and youth. A support program for HIV-infected women aims at prevention of perinatal transmission. Communication of educational services to agencies and groups provides education to youth, particularly those who are at risk for contracting HIV. The project's approach involves case managers, the interdisciplinary team, educational networks, clients and their families, family support workers, foster parents, and trained volunteers. Evaluation has been designed to track activities and to measure achievement based on project goals.[50]

Another program, the Curriculum Development for Training Family Service Providers, teaches people to work with families of HIV-infected children. Its goals include developing a training program, recruiting conference participants, conducting a workshop, expanding the model to other training curriculums, and improving services to children with HIV infection.[51]

The Compassionate Friends Organization in Oak Brook, Illinois, is designed to educate families, teachers, and the general public about children with AIDS. The group provides guidelines for parents and children on such issues as dealing with the truth, being aware of feelings, and forming relationships between adults and children. The group's work with teachers consists of suggestions on how to treat with patience children who have short attention spans, learning about the child's concept of death, teaching children that death is a natural part of life, encouraging feeling, and being aware of a child's need for time alone.[52]

The Palliative Care Center for Children in Bayside, New York, works to provide expert medical care for pain control, meet child and family needs, help both to understand the child's condition, give support during times of stress, and continue support and comfort to the family after the child's death. The program offers home care, day care, and inpatient care. Children may enjoy music, recreation, lounges, terraces, an attractive skylight, and a beautiful view of Little Neck Bay. The team consists of physicians, nurses, social workers, therapists, clergy, and volunteers; services in psychology, pharmacology, nutrition, dentistry, and education are provided. The program accepts children under sixteen years of age and can be financed through Medicaid or private insurance.[53]

Helen House was developed through a relationship that a critically ill girl named Helen had with Mother Frances Dominica, founder and director of Helen House. Today, Helen House is used by 120 families from all over the country; they take children and adolescents up to age twenty. Their objective is to support parents and families who are facing the tragedy of incurable and life-threatening illness in their children.[54]

The Hospice of St. John, a nongovernmental hospice organization, is a fully accredited and licensed care facility providing care and support to the terminally ill of all ages. It is a nonprofit institution, which employs a licensed administrator, a medical director, four medical residents, a twenty-four-hour skilled care team, a pastoral staff, a bereavement team, and volunteers.[55]

Located in Daytona Beach, Florida, the Hospice of Volusia/ Flager is also a nongovernmental hospice organization. It provides services in counseling, medical and home nursing care, finance, and homemaking. These services are available to adults with AIDS, children with AIDS, and infants with AIDS.[56]

The Hospice of Northeast Florida is another nongovernmental hospice organization located in Jacksonville. Spiritual and pastoral counseling, funeral services, medical services, home nursing care, and other hospice services are included. These are available to children, families, friends, adults with AIDS, and children with AIDS.[57]

Hospice Incorporated is a nongovernmental hospice program that provides services to adults with AIDS, children with AIDS, and any HIV-infected person. Counseling services, medical services, educational services, and information dissemination services are offered in English, Spanish, and Haitian languages.[58]

St. Joseph's Hospital, a nongovernmental hospice organization in Fort Worth, Texas, provides spiritual and pastoral counseling, funeral assistance, home nursing care, home health aides, and library services. This hospice serves health professionals, community service professionals, the general public, families and friends of AIDS patients, persons with AIDS, children with AIDS, intravenous drug users, HIV-infected people, and community organizations.[59]

CONCLUSION

In September 1990, the World Health Organization (WHO) analyzed the AIDS epidemic. WHO concluded that AIDS would be the major cause of death in the 1990s. In some countries, it will be the number one cause of death for infants and children. Worldwide, an estimated three million women of childbearing age are infected with HIV.[60] It is clear that these numbers are increasing.

With the number of pediatric AIDS cases rapidly increasing, health professionals need to be familiar with all aspects of HIV infection. They must acquaint themselves with the medical and psychosocial implications of the disease. Team work is necessary in caring for the infected child. The hospice program can be very beneficial in helping the dying child and his or her family through the dying process and the many complications and problems that may arise with this disease. By adopting the holistic approach of hospice, the diverse needs of the pediatric AIDS patients and their families can be met.

NOTES

1. World Health Organization, "In Point of Fact," May 1991, p. 1.

2. A. Meyers and M. Weitzman, "Pediatric HIV Disease: The Newest Chronic Illness of Childhood," *Pediatric Clinics of North America* 38 (1991): 169.

3. J. Zylke, "Another Consequence of Uncontrolled Spread of HIV Among Adults: Vertical Transmission," *Journal of the American Medical Association* 265 (1991): 1798.

4. P. Pizzo, "Pediatric AIDS: Problems within Problems," *The Journal of Infectious Diseases* 161 (1990): 316.

5. Ibid., pp. 317–18.

6. Task Force on Pediatric AIDS, "Pediatric AIDS and Human Immunodeficiency Virus Infection: Psychological Issues," *American Psychologist* (1989): 258.

7. N. Karthas and S. Chancock, "Clinical Management of HIV-Infection in Infants and Children," *Family Community Health* 13 (1990): 8.

8. L. Lockhart and J. Wodarski, "Facing the Unknown: Children and Adolescents with AIDS," *Social Work* (1989): 217.

9. U.S. Department of Education, *AIDS and the Education of Our Children: A Guide for Parents and Teachers* (Washington, D.C., 1987).

10. R. J. DiClemente, T. Zorn, and L. Temoshok, "Adolescents and AIDS: A Survey of Knowledge, Attitudes, and Beliefs about AIDS in San Francisco," *American Journal of Public Health* 76 (1986): 1443–45.

11. Lockhart and Wodarski, "Facing the Unknown: Children and Adolescents with AIDS," p. 217.

12. Centers for Disease Control, "Recommendations for Prevention of HIV Transmission in Health-Care Settings," *Morbidity and Mortality Weekly Report* 36, suppl. 2 (1987): 3–18.

13. M. F. Rogers, "AIDS in Children: A Review of the Clinical Epidemiologic and Public Health Aspects," *Pediatric Infectious Disease* 4 (1985): 230–36.

14. J. Oleske, "Natural History of HIV Infection II," in *Report*

of the Surgeon General's Workshop on Children with HIV Infection and Their Families, K. B. Silverman and A. Waddell, eds. (Washington, D.C.: U.S. Department of Health and Human Services, 1987), pp. 24–25.

15. Department of Health, State of New York, *AIDS—Get the Facts!* (Albany, N.Y.).

16. Lockhart and Wodarski, "Facing the Unknown: Children and Adolescents with AIDS," p. 217.

17. E. Chachkes, "Women and Children with AIDS," in *Responding to AIDS: Psychosocial Initiatives,* C. Leukefeld and M. Fimbres, eds. (Silver Spring, Md.: National Association of Social Workers, 1987), pp. 51–64.

18. National Institute of Mental Health, *Coping with AIDS: Psychological and Social Considerations in Helping Pelple with HTLV-III Infection* (Rockville, Md., 1986).

19. M. L. Belfer, "Psychological Impact of AIDS on Children," *Viewpoints* 120 (1986): 2–29.

20. Chachkes, "Women and Children with AIDS," pp. 51–64.

21. J. Smakulowich, "Adolescents Face Up to AIDS," *AIDS Patient Care* (1988): 38.

22. Task Force on Pediatric AIDS, "Pediatric AIDS and Human Immunodeficiency Virus Infection: Psychological Issues," p. 259.

23. M. L. Belfer, "Psychological Impact of AIDS on Children," pp. 2–29.

24. Chachkes, "Women and Children with AIDS," pp. 51–64.

25. G. A. Anderson, *Children and AIDS: The Challenge for Child Welfare* (Washington, D.C.: Child Welfare League of America, 1986).

26. C. Lewin and R. J. W. Williams, "Fear of AIDS: The Impact of Public Anxiety in Young People," *British Journal of Psychiatrics* 153 (1988): 823.

27. Ibid., pp. 823–24.

28. Ibid., p. 824.

29. Smakulowich, "Adolescents Face Up to AIDS," p. 39.

30. A. Armstrong-Dailey, "Children's Hospice Care," *Pediatric Nursing* 16 (1990): 339.

31. Ibid., p. 338.

32. A. Armstrong-Dailey, "Program Organization Chart," *Caring* (1989): 26.

33. A. Parker, "Hospice Care: An Untapped Resource," *AIDS Patient Care* (1988): 37.

34. C. Clark et al. "Hospice Care: A Model for Caring for the Person with AIDS," *Nursing Clinics of North America* 23 (1988): 852.

35. B. Rusnack, S. McNulty Schaefer, and D. Moxley, " 'Safe Passage': Social Work Roles and Functions in Hospice Care," *Social Work and Health Care* 13 (1988): 6.

36. Task Force on Pediatric AIDS, "Pediatric AIDS and Human Immunodeficiency Virus Infection," p. 259.

37. H. O'Connor, "Recruiting and Training Volunteers," *Caring* (1990): 54.

38. Rusnack et al., " 'Safe Passage': Social Work Roles and Functions in Hospice Care," p. 6.

39. "Guidelines for the Protection of Health Care Workers in Caring for Persons Who Have Some Form of HTLV-III/LAV Infection," *New York Journal of Medicine* 86 (11): 587-91.

40. C. Betz and E. Poster, "Children's Concepts of Death," *Nursing Clinics of North America* 19 (1984): 342-44.

41. L. Spiegal and A. Mayers, "Psychosocial Aspects of AIDS in Children and Adolescents," *Pediatric Clinics of North America* 38 (1990): 156-57.

42. R. Buckingham, *Care of the Dying Child* (New York, N.Y.: Continuum, 1989), pp. 56-58.

43. A. Miles, "Caring for Families When a Child Dies," *Pediatric Nursing* 16 (1990): 247.

44. E. Katz, "Talking with Dying Children," *Pediatric Hospice Conference Report* (1985): 57-58.

45. M. Pizzi, "Occupational Therapy: Creating Possibilities for Children with HIV-Infection, ARC, and AIDS," *AIDS Patient Care* (1989): 31-36.

46. Y. Williams, "Symbolic Expressions of Body and Soul in Children's Art," *Pediatric Hospice Conference Report* (1985): 69-70.

47. Betz and Poster, "Children's Concepts of Death," p. 341.

48. Buckingham, *Care of the Dying Child,* p. 67.

49. B. McIntyre, "An Art Therapy Group for Bereaved Youth in Hospice Care," *Caring* (1990): 56–58.

50. *Pediatric AIDS: Abstracts of Active Projects FY 1990 and FY 1991* (Washington, D.C.: National Center for Education in Maternal and Child Health, 1991), pp. 58–59.

51. Ibid., pp. 51–52.

52. *Caring for Surviving Children* (Oak Brook, Ill.: The Compassionate Friends, Inc.).

53. *There Is a Time for Wishing and for Many Wishes to Come True* (Bayside, N.Y.: Palliative Care Center, St. Mary's Hospital for Children, Inc.).

54. M. Dominica, "Helen House: A Hospice for Children," *Pediatric Hospice Conference Report* (1985): 15–22.

55. *Hospice of St. John* (Washington, D.C.: National AIDS Information Clearing House).

56. Ibid.

57. Ibid.

58. Ibid.

59. Ibid.

60. Centers for Disease Control, "AIDS Predicted to Be the Major Cause of Pediatric Death in the 1990s," *Caring* (1990): 40–41.

7

The Cost of Care for Persons with AIDS
Mary Derby

INTRODUCTION

By 1993, the total number of reported cases of Acquired Immuno-deficiency Syndrome (AIDS) in the United States is expected to reach 480,000. It is estimated that approximately one million Americans are currently infected with the human immunodeficiency virus (HIV). Each year, according to the Centers for Disease Control (CDC), 40,000 new infections occur among adults and adolescents, and an estimated 1,500 to 2,000 new infections occur each year among newborns as a result of perinatal HIV transmission. It is predicted that most of the individuals infected with HIV will eventually become ill and require care. The current and future cost of care for persons with AIDS (PWAs) and HIV infection continues to be of great concern.

AIDS affects primarily young adults in their twenties, thirties, and forties. To date, homosexual men have accounted for 55 percent of reported U.S. AIDS cases. However, the number of cases is increasing among intravenous (IV)-drug abusers, minorities, and infants.[1] Increasing numbers of homeless PWAs have been noted, particularly among those who are IV-drug abusers. With no cure yet for AIDS or even a viable vaccine, most individuals die within two years of initial diagnosis. Treatment for persons with AIDS has typically occurred in acute hospital settings. This is very costly, and places a strain on the capacity of hospitals in the areas most heavily affected.[2]

Increasingly it has been recognized that AIDS patients could be treated in alternative settings. People with AIDS in the terminal stages of the illness could benefit from hospice services; hospice, with its emphasis on palliative and supportive care, is an appropriate and cost-effective alternative to the acute hospital setting. There are a variety of settings where hospice care can be provided to meet each individual PWA's needs.

GENERAL COSTS

Over the past few years, researchers have attempted to estimate the medical care cost of persons with AIDS. These estimates have varied considerably depending on the definition of AIDS used, the scope and definition of costs, and the time period and geographic area studied.[3] The initial report on the cost of treating PWAs by the Public Health Service's Centers for Disease Control in 1985 forecasted a cost of $147,000 per AIDS patient from initial diagnosis until death. This estimate was based on 168 inpatient days and an average survival time of about thirteen months.[4] Subsequent studies reflect much lower lifetime medical care costs and reduced hospital stays. Recent estimates of the lifetime medical care costs per PWA, from diagnosis to death, have ranged from between $55,000 and $80,000,[5] with estimates of between $50,000 and $60,000 considered most likely.[6] Approximately 90 percent of the medical care costs of persons with AIDS have been related to use of inpatient services.[7] On average, AIDS patients require between 1.6 and 3.5 hospitalizations per year, with average lengths of stay ranging from 15 to 25 days.[8]

National medical care costs for persons with AIDS for 1991

have been estimated to be $8.5 billion.[9] This figure, representing 1.4 percent of the total personal health care expenditures for 1991— up from 0.2 percent in 1985—is less than the cost of treating other serious illnesses.

These estimates, however, do not provide a complete picture of the cost of care for persons with AIDS. Many studies have excluded non-hospital costs such as drugs, ambulatory and ancillary services, long-term care, hospice and home health care, counseling, and other community services. There are limited data available on the use and costs of medical care for IV-drug abusers, women, and pediatric patients. In addition, much less is known about the costs incurred by HIV-infected individuals who have not yet developed AIDS. As a result of these shortcomings, the cost estimates to date most likely underestimate the full economic impact of AIDS.

THE COST OF AIDS: SOME PRELIMINARY CONSIDERATIONS

Total costs associated with AIDS,* including both direct and indirect costs, have been estimated to reach $66.5 billion in 1991, of which $56 billion, or approximately 84 percent, represents indirect costs.[10] Indirect costs reflect the losses incurred as a result of the disability or premature death of working-age adults. These costs could rise even higher in the future: transmission of the virus has not yet peaked, and the percentage of HIV-infected individuals who will develop AIDS continues to increase.[11]

The medical management of AIDS care has changed and will continue to change over time, although whether this will lower or raise medical care costs presently remains unclear. There are reports that AIDS patients are less likely now to be admitted to intensive

---

*Cost studies for people with AIDS vary widely. The findings almost always refer to lifetime medical costs. However, one study by Seage et al. (1986) reported an average hospital cost of $14,189 based on an average of 1.6 hospitalizations per year, and average length of stay of twenty-one days per hospitalization. The researchers calculated the average cost per patient per year at $46,505 and cost per patient, from initial diagnosis to death, at $50,380.

care units than they were earlier and that the average length of hospital stay has declined.[12] A reduction in hospital use has been attributed to alternative models of health care delivery which rely on outpatient care and community-based services. The cost of these services will need to be evaluated in order to analyze the cost implications of relying less on hospitalizations and more on community support services.[13]

The introduction of new treatment modalities will also influence costs. One such example is the widespread use of zidovudine (AZT). AZT has been found to decrease the incidence of life-threatening pneumonia in persons with AIDS, which may ultimately reduce medical costs by eliminating or shortening lengths of hospitalization. Alternatively, AZT may increase treatment costs. It is an expensive drug (costing between $8,000 and $10,000 per patient per year) and requires close medical monitoring. As many as 30 percent of AIDS patients on AZT may develop severe anemia and require regular blood transfusions. Although AZT appears to increase the life expectancy of AIDS sufferers, they may still die from other AIDS-related disorders, such as dementia, which can be even more expensive.[14]

Because complications resulting from AIDS appear to differ among high-risk groups, changes in incidence patterns could influence the cost of the disease.[15] Early in the epidemic, the majority of AIDS cases were homosexual or bisexual males; but now the trend is changing, with an increasing proportion of IV-drug abusers, women, minorities, and children being noted.[16] These changes in the demographic profile of people with AIDS will have a dramatic effect on health resources and medical costs in certain metropolitan areas.[17] For example, more than 75 percent of the U.S. AIDS cases in which patients contracted the disease through IV-drug use have been in New York City.[18] Forty percent of the nation's pediatric AIDS cases have also occurred there.[19] The costs associated with caring for people with AIDS who are IV-drug abusers and children with AIDS are considered to be higher and more likely to be social than medical.[20] Oftentimes these patients remain in an acute care setting longer because they have no one to care for them, or else they do not have a suitable place to go when they are discharged.

Changes in the geographic distribution of the AIDS population may also have an impact on the costs of care. What sort of impact is difficult to predict. In the early stages of the epidemic, New York and San Francisco accounted for 34 percent of U.S. AIDS cases, but as the epidemic has continued to spread, it has diminished to 20 percent. Thus the impact has resulted in a shift to smaller urban centers that may not have health care delivery systems adequately equipped to provide the care most people with AIDS need.[21] Additionally it has been found that hospital costs are lower in the West than the Northeast, and that these variations are caused by differences in the average length of hospital stay (24 days in the Northeast versus 14 days in the West). Differences in patient diagnosis appear to explain most of the variation in length of hospitalization. The incidence of IV-drug abusers with AIDS is higher in the Northeast, thus accounting for longer lengths of stay and more days per year than in the West.[22]

Finally, in addition to the uncertainties about overall costs per se, there are growing concerns regarding where the funding for care will come from. Recent studies demonstrate a shift from private to public financing, with 40 percent of all people with AIDS being served under the Medicaid program. In states like New York and New Jersey, the proportion may be as high as 65 percent to 70 percent.[23] The Health Care Financing Administration (HCFA) has estimated that Medicaid spending for AIDS care, excluding the cost of AZT, would be some $2.4 billion by 1992. The estimated cost alone of providing AZT will exceed $120 million.[24] Even so, there are concerns that Medicaid coverage is inadequate to meet most individuals' needs. States have flexibility in determining which services they will reimburse; this may mean that some states are meeting the needs of persons with AIDS more effectively than others.[25] Additionally there has been concern regarding the impact this will have on state finances and on the Medicaid program in general.[26] As more money is allocated for AIDS care, Medicaid coverage for other groups could be restricted.

The increasing numbers of AIDS cases and the cost associated with new treatment modalities will undoubtedly place a tremendous burden on the health care delivery system as it currently exists. To date, medical management of the illness has been primarily in the inpatient setting. This is not only costly, but often medically unnecessary. Many times AIDS patients remain in acute settings, when there is no medical need, because of the lack of appropriate alternatives.[27] In order to reduce the cost of care for persons with AIDS, effective alternatives to hospitalization will need to be utilized.

The progression of the AIDS illness varies for each patient. Some individuals die soon after diagnosis. For others, the illness is chronic with periods of acute illness, interspersed with long periods of relative stability during which time they may be able to work. Most persons with AIDS will require inpatient hospital services at some point during the course of their illness. The rest of the time they can be maintained at home with home care services. Other people with AIDS, particularly those suffering from AIDS dementia complex, may require institutional care. People with AIDS in the terminal stage of the illness could benefit from hospice services.

Many communities are developing comprehensive care systems similar to San Francisco's approach, which combines acute hospital AIDS treatment units with community services. This system is considered to be the most effective approach to providing care to the person with AIDS over the course of the illness. San Francisco utilizes a continuum-of-care model, which includes a designated hospital AIDS unit, a hospital-based outpatient clinic, and a comprehensive network of home and community-based services.[28] Lifetime medical care costs for AIDS patients in San Francisco have been lower than in other areas of the country as a result of fewer hospitalizations and shorter lengths of stay.[29] This experience has been widely attributed to the effective use of community-based services such as home care, hospice, and support services. Additionally, San Francisco utilizes a network of trained volunteers who assist patients with meal preparation, light housework, transportation to clinic appointments; or who provide relief to caregivers.

Three major concerns must be addressed before hospice gains wider acceptance as an alternative to current treatment by people with AIDS and their families, hospice providers, and the public: (1) defining and determining a market for hospice, (2) demonstrating cost effectiveness of hospice care compared to current alternatives, and (3) assuring third-party reimbursement for hospice care.

HOSPICE AS AN ALTERNATIVE: SOME WORKING MODELS

Over the past decade, the use of hospice services has moved into the mainstream of cancer care. Legislation passed by Congress in 1982 provided for ongoing federal reimbursement for hospice and was predicated on the assumption that hospice care for dying patients resulted in lower health care costs.[30] Since 1982, Medicaid and other third-party payers such as Blue Cross/Blue Shield have also been providing reimbursement for hospice services.

AIDS is similar to cancer and other terminal illnesses in that hospitalizations are most frequent in the early and late stages of the illness.[31] Thus, as with other terminally ill patients, reduced costs for persons with AIDS can be achieved by providing more relevant palliative care in lieu of hospital services during the final months of life. The hospice service package includes: pain and symptom control, pastoral/spiritual counseling, bereavement services for patients and their families, twenty-four-hour on-call nurse/counselor, and respite for caregivers. These services have been effective for other terminally ill patients, and are equally suitable for people with AIDS and their families. Hospice teams can utilize their present knowledge related to symptom management, death and dying, and bereavement needs of family and friends to expand their programs for the terminally ill person with AIDS.

San Francisco

As noted above, hospice services have been utilized by AIDS patients in San Francisco as an alternative to hospitalization since the early stages of the epidemic. Evidence of this is the expansion of Shanti, a hospice organization that, prior to the AIDS epidemic, gave help and emotional support to terminally ill patients, and that now provides its services almost exclusively to people with AIDS.[32] It appears that the demand for these services is growing. The AIDS Home Care and Hospice Program in San Francisco increased its daily caseload from eighteen patients initially to 63 patients in 1986, with a waiting list of 30 to 45 patients.[33] Over 90 percent of AIDS cases served by this program have died at home, while 10 percent have died in a hospital or have been discharged from the program when hospice services were no longer needed.

San Francisco's experience demonstrates that a market for home hospice services for persons with AIDS exists and is best suited for individuals who have a supportive network of friends and family available to assist with their care. Some terminally ill patients, however, cannot be maintained at home because they do not have friends or family available to assist with their care, or because they do not have a place to live. In such situations the patient requires residential care or housing.[34] Hospice programs are now developing creative approaches to meet the needs of these individuals by providing their services to people with AIDS who are living in group homes, or in some instances developing their own residential hospice facility to meet the needs of terminally ill AIDS patients in their community.

Cambridge, Massachusetts

Hospice of Cambridge, Inc. will soon be opening the first home hospice in Massachusetts. It will be operated and licensed as a boarding home. Although this home is not specifically for people with AIDS, it is an example of a hospice program providing a unique cost-effective and humane option for the terminally ill. The hospice provider vigorously pursued sources of funding, and acquired and renovated a house to provide a residence where terminally ill homeless patients and those who could no longer be supported in their home would be able to receive hospice services. This home will accommodate up to five residents and has additional space for children and significant others. It will be staffed by a full-time residential manager and two full-time attendants. Residents will pay for room and board on a sliding scale, and their insurance company will be billed at the routine hospice home care rate. The cost of care for those served by this program will be the same as the cost of home-based hospice services. This not only provides a cost-effective service, but, more important, will enhance the quality of life for the patients being served during the final stages of their illness.

Residential hospice facilities that are often associated with existing hospice home care programs are also being utilized to care for the terminally ill person with AIDS. These facilities were designed to provide a greater intensity of services within a home-like atmosphere for the patient. These facilities are suitable for the terminally ill who can no longer be maintained at home because of inadequate support systems or for individuals who require a significant amount of skilled nursing or attendant care. They provide an ideal setting for the person with AIDS who is exhibiting cognitive impairments, ranging from short-term memory loss to full dementia resembling Alzheimer's and requiring twenty-four-hour supervision in advanced stages. These residential facilities are reimbursed at the Medicare/Medicaid established inpatient hospice rate, or through negotiated rates with third-party payers. This rate is higher than the routine home care rate, but much less than the rate of acute hospitalization.

The group home residence model and the inpatient residential facility are two examples of the way hospice programs have adapted their services to meet the needs of the terminally ill AIDS patient. However, the extent to which hospice programs will be able further to expand their services will depend on acceptance of the hospice philosophy by persons with AIDS and their families. Some people with AIDS may not be ready to accept palliative care only, and may choose to seek aggressive therapy for each opportunistic infection. With AIDS affecting primarily a younger population, the introduction of new therapies provides hope for survival despite the predicted short life expectancies. Therefore, hospice programs that can be flexible and allow the use of experimental drugs or provide services to individuals living alone wll be more attractive to people with AIDS.[35]

THE COST OF HOSPICE CARE VERSUS HOSPITALIZATION

The next area of concern for hospice care is that of demonstrating its cost effectiveness compared to standard available alternatives. Very few studies have analyzed the cost effectiveness of services enabling AIDS patients to remain at home and out of institutions for as long as possible.[36] Only one study to date has evaluated the cost effectiveness of a home-based hospice program for people with AIDS. Although the results were positive, the study looked at patients residing in one geographic area only. It needs to be determined whether or not these results can be duplicated elsewhere.

Research studies on the cost effectiveness of hospice care for terminally ill cancer patients have generally been encouraging: savings have resulted from substituting less costly home care for acute care during the final months of life.[37] One striking example of such savings appeared in a study comparing the costs of the last two weeks of life for patients dying in the hospital versus those dying at home. The study found hospital costs to be 10.5 times greater than home care costs, the higher cost being attributable to the greater use of diagnostic and therapeutic services.[38]

A study by Mor and Kidder[39] found similar results. They compared the costs of both home care and hospital-based hospice programs to those of conventional care for terminal cancer patients. The greatest savings were noted in the last month of life. The cost of treatment for conventional care patients was nearly three times as high as that of home care hospice patients. Overall costs for the last year of life were lower for home care and hospital-based hospice patients than for their conventional care counterparts. Again, the difference in costs was attributed to the substitution of home care services for inpatient care and a reduction in the intensity of ancillary service use for hospital-based hospice patients.*

A San Francisco study evaluating the effectiveness of a home-based hospice program for people with AIDS found it to be far less expensive than inpatient hospitalization.[40] The study found that the 165 AIDS patients who received hospice care from this program during fiscal year 1985 required an average of 47 hospice days per person at an average per diem cost per patient of $94, for a total cost per patient of $4,401. Although this was not a randomized controlled study, the implications for cost savings are great when compared to the costs to AIDS patients of treatment at San Francisco General Hospital. There the average per diem cost was $773; the

---

*For more detail on this study, see Appendix B.

average cost per hospitalization, $9,024; and the total lifetime cost for patients who received all their care at San Francisco General Hospital, $27,571.[41] Additional data from San Francisco estimate the cost of available alternatives to home-based hospice for people with AIDS to be much higher. Chen's study, as cited in Landers and Seage, estimated the average cost of acute inpatient care at $800 a day; subacute care at $500 a day; a skilled nursing facility at $300 a day; and a residential hospice at $100 a day.[42] These comparisons further demonstrate the magnitude of the cost effectiveness of home-based hospice programs.

Alternatives to acute hospitalization for terminally ill AIDS patients include any of the following: home care, home-based hospice care, hospice care provided in a group home or inpatient residential facility, or institutional care in either chronic hospitals or skilled nursing facilities. Any of these settings are appropriate and needed in order to prevent people with AIDS from being hospitalized in acute care settings. The most appropriate setting for any terminally ill AIDS patient will depend on his or her care needs, home environment, social support network, insurance coverage, and community setting.[43] Because of the nature of the illness, any one of these settings may be appropriate for a person with AIDS at any given time.

For individuals who require twenty-four-hour care and who cannot be maintained at home, placement in a hospice inpatient residential facility or an institutional setting becomes necessary. Although the availability and cost of such options will depend on the community where the patient resides, a sound estimate of the cost of a chronic care hospital is $500 a day; an inpatient residential hospice facility, $350 a day; and care in a skilled nursing facility can range from $125 to $200 a day. Still, all these options are far less expensive than an acute care facility, where costs can range from $800 to $1,000 a day. Anecdotal evidence suggests that most people with AIDS would prefer to remain at home or in noninstitutional settings rather than in hospitals or nursing homes.[44] While the lower cost of a nursing home may make it appear to be a more desirable alternative, experience to date has demonstrated a reluctance by both AIDS patients and nursing homes to accept this option. People with AIDS prefer to be in a home-like environment and with individuals who are closer to their own age. There are a number of reasons why nursing homes have not been used. The current high occupancy rate in nursing homes enables administrators to select the patients they wish to admit. Many nursing homes do not have the staffing capacity and are concerned about the additional cost of providing the physical and psychosocial care AIDS patients would require. Current nursing home rates are already considered to be inadequate by the industry.[45]

Home-based hospice services can be utilized by the terminally ill AIDS patient who prefers to remain at home. Most programs will provide services to those who live alone as long as they have someone who can be available to help if needed. This alternative is not only cost-effective but provides such services as attendant care, volunteer support, bereavement counseling, and twenty-four-hour on-call nurse coverage, which are all critically needed to maintain the patient at home.

Hospice services will not be acceptable to all terminally ill AIDS patients; some will continue to seek treatment aimed at cure, even when home-bound. These patients can receive home care services offered by a visiting nurse association. Both programs provide similar services and are often combined within a single agency. However, there is an important distinction between these two types of services. Home care services are aimed at treatment of acute problems, with the individual being the unit of care. Insurers will reimburse skilled care only, and as such will not reimburse for social work services or bereavement counseling. Hospice services encompass both the physical and emotional needs of the individual and are provided to the entire family.

Case Study

"Michael," a twenty-seven-year-old married man with two children ages two and five, was admitted to a hospice program after discharge from the hospital. Michael was diagnosed with AIDS and myco-bacterium avium intracellulare (MAI) approximately one year earlier, and prior to admission had been maintained at home with the support of home care services. Over the past year he had received intermittent skilled nursing visits to monitor medication compliance, nutritional status, and blood work.

Michael was hospitalized for treatment of Pneumocystis pneumonia (PCP), malnutrition, and anemia secondary to use of AZT. Despite treatment, his physical status continued to deteriorate. Recognizing that treatment was no longer working, Michael requested to be discharged so that he could be at home with his wife and children. He had been hospitalized for 54 days, with total charges amounting to $60,090.02, or approximately $1,113 a day.

A nurse and social worker from the hospice program made the first visit together. The nurse assessed Michael's physical care needs, and arranged for daily home health aide services to assist with bathing and ambulation. The social worker discussed Michael's concerns with him. Michael had not been able to pay his rent and had just received an eviction notice; his wife had not been able to work because she had no one to assist with child care.

The social worker spoke with the landlord and arranged to have the family stay in the apartment for one more month. The hospice program paid the rent with donations for that month, while the social worker continued to look for housing. The social worker consulted with the AIDS coordinator at e local AIDS service organization, who found subsidized housing for the family. The hospice program provided family counseling and child care through volunteers. Michael's status steadily improved; after two months he was discharged from the program as services were no longer needed. Michael has been receiving biweekly nursing visits for administration of medications. He is no longer home-bound and has remained out of the hospital for the past six months.

This case study highlights several important points about the appropriateness of hospice care for terminally ill AIDS patients. First, it demonstrates the commitment of a hospice program to assess fully and to provide all of the individual's needs. In this case, the hospice program was well integrated into the community and was able to access volunteers and resources from other agencies. Second, it demonstrates the unpredictable course of the AIDS illness. Michael was considered to be in the terminal stages of the disease; however, his prognosis improved quite dramatically without curative treatment. Whether or not this can be attributed to hospice services is unclear; but the hospice program was able to remove the significant stress factors from Michael's life. As a result, Michael was able to concentrate all his energies on himself. Third, the cost effectiveness of hospice services for this individual were significant. The cost of home-based hospice care is less than $100 a day, which is less costly by far than care in an inpatient or chronic care facility. Additionally, Michael has remained out of an acute care facility for six months. Finally, this case study demonstrates the useful application of two different home care services. Hospice, with its integrated network of resources and services aimed at palliative care, was more suitable than home care services during the terminal stages. Home care services were effective when Michael required only skilled care.

Another major concern to be discussed in hospice care for the terminally ill person with AIDS is third-party reimbursement. Private insurers concerned about the high costs of medical care for people with AIDS are increasingly willing to reimburse for optional services that can be demonstrated to be both cost-effective and appropriate alternatives to hospitalization for their clients. Hospice care is an optional benefit, therefore, which most insurance policies cover. Typically, insurance companies case-manage clients on an individual basis, and review alternative treatment plans submitted by hospital discharge planners or social workers in community agencies. The insurer will reimburse the alternative service requested, if it can be demonstated to be cost-effective. The following is an alternative treatment plan developed by a hospital discharge planner and submitted to the patient's insurance company.

Case Study

"John" is a thirty-six-year-old man in the terminal stages of AIDS, who is currently hospitalized in an acute care facility. Over the course of his hospitalization John has received treatment for PCP, cytomegalovirus (CMV), oral thrush, malnutrition, and dehydration. John has made the decision to cease curative care. He is now ready for discharge pending approval of appropriate placement. John requires long-term placement for twenty-four-hour attendant care and administration of intravenous DHPG (ganciclovir) to prevent blindness secondary to CMV. John is confined to bed. He has frequent episodes of explosive diarrhea. He is too weak to feed or bathe himself. Because of John's care needs, he cannot be maintained at home. Discharge would normally be to a chronic care facility where his acute care needs can be met. However, John has requested to be transferred to an inpatient residence hospice facility in his community.

The sole purpose of this alternative treatment plan is to cover the cost of the patient's admission to an inpatient hospice facility that is Medicare-approved and state-licensed. The daily cost will be $380 inclusive of medications. This fee includes twenty-four-hour skilled nursing care, room and board, and any durable medical equipment the patient may require. Based on a seven-day week, the estimated cost will be $2,660 a week or $10,640 a month. John will also receive intravenous DHPG (gamma cyclovere) three times a week at an estimated cost of $70 per dose. Estimated weekly costs will be $210 a day or $840 a month. The combined estimated monthly cost will then amount to $11,480.00.

Total charges to date at the acute care facility are $67,979.40, based on 46 hospital days, or $1,477.81 a day. It is anticipated that the patient would have been routinely admitted to a chronic care facility at an estimated cost of $566.67 a day, $4,250 a week, and $17,000 a month. The alternative treatment plan requests transfer to an inpatient residential hospice facility, which reflects an estimated cost savings of $1,380 a week or $4,520 a month. After review of the alternative treatment plan, the insurance company approved transfer to the inpatient residential hospice.

This case demonstrates the high cost of hospital care for persons with AIDS during the terminal stages of the illness. It is not uncommon for people with AIDS to continue to seek aggressive treatment aimed at cure for as long as possible. Additionally, some AIDS patients may need to remain in very costly acute care facilities because of the lack of appropriate alternatives. This case also demonstrates the willingness of third-party payers to negotiate rates with hospice providers, thereby ensuring adequate reimbursement. This patient's care needs were such that he could not be maintained at home. If home hospice care was an appropriate alternative, the cost savings would have been much greater. The cost of home hospice care is less than $100 a day, which is dramatically less than the cost of chronic care.

Finally, there is anecdotal evidence that Medicare and Medicaid's reimbursement rates may not be adequate to cover the cost of care for the terminally ill AIDS patient. These rates were designed to cover the cost of caring for the terminally ill cancer patient. The cost of providing care for people with AIDS is often high as a result of increased costs for medications and attendant care. The cost of medications for cancer patients averages $10 to $15 a day, while the costs of medications for people with AIDS averages $45 a day. Hospice providers are reimbursed by Medicare and Medicaid at a per diem all-inclusive rate, and as such are unable to bill separately for medications or equipment. If John had been a Medicaid recipient, the hospice program would have had to absorb the $210 weekly cost of providing DHPG to the patient. Frequently the person with AIDS, because of neurologic impairments, requires between eight and twenty-four hours per day of attendant care. Based on current reimbursement rates, hospice programs can only provide up to twenty hours of attendant care per client per week. Hospice programs often substitute volunteer care when possible; however, if the AIDS patient requires skilled care, they will provide the additional coverage and absorb the extra cost.

The high cost of caring for people with AIDS within Medicare and Medicaid's present reimbursement structure could place a strain on hospice providers. Medicaid currently covers the cost of care for 40 percent of all people with AIDS. It is anticipated that in future years this could increase, depending on future epidemiologic trends, in particular, the spread of HIV infection among intravenous drug abusers.[46] Given the implications of this, Medicaid's rates may need to be enhanced to encourage hospice programs to serve AIDS patients insured by this program. A precedent for this has already been established. The Omnibus Budget Reconciliation Act of 1987 permitted waivers of the inpatient care limitations for Medicare and Medicaid hospice patients with AIDS.[47] Normally hospice providers are penalized if patients are treated on an inpatient basis more than 20 percent of the time. This waiver prevents hospice providers from being penalized for AIDS patients who use up their inpatient limits; however, people with AIDS continue to be subject to overall per-patient dollar limits. To ensure more equitable reimbursement, hospice providers could be allowed to bill Medicare and Medicaid for medications on a fee-for-service basis in addition to the per diem rates. This would relieve the burden of some of the costs, and still be a more cost-effective alternative than care in an acute or chronic care facility.

SUMMARY

Hospice, with its emphasis on coordinated care, including intensive home care, counseling, and support services, is one viable option along a continuum of care which should be offered to terminally ill AIDS patients. Support for these services appears to be increasing among people with AIDS. Many, however, are not ready to accept the terminal status of the illness. Although there is no cure to date, the introduction of new treatments has prompted many persons with AIDS to continue to seek aggressive medical treatment.

The costs associated with medical care for people with AIDS are high. Concern over the increasing numbers of AIDS patients who will require services and the subsequent strain this could place on the current health system has prompted expansion of alternative settings to acute and chronic hospital care. Hospice has been demonstrated to be an appropriate and cost-effective alternative to hospital care for the terminally ill AIDS patient. With its broad service package, hospice care can be provided in many different settings to meet the needs of the person with AIDS. Many hospice providers have already developed innovative programs for people with AIDS.

APPENDIX A

Personal Medical Care Costs Associated with AIDS

If independent information on life expectancy is not reported in a study, we assume a period of thirteen months if needed to calculate lifetime costs.[48] "Life expectancy" refers to the period following an AIDS diagnosis, except in Kizer et al.;[49] "days" refers to the average number of days hospitalized following an AIDS diagnosis, unless otherwise indicated; "charge or cost per day" is average medical charge or cost (as indicated) per inpatient day. NA, not applicable.

Background Information	Life expectancy	Days	Personal medical care costs (1986 dollars)		
			Charge or cost per day	Per case over lifetime	Cumulative total to end of 1991
Costs from 169 metropolitan public and private teaching hospitals with 5,393 AIDS patients during 1985.[50]	NA	34	683*	23,000*	6.3 billion*
Hospital cost data for 26 Baltimore AIDS patients hospitalized between 1979 and February 1985 who had died by the time of the study.[51]	24 weeks	50	723*	36,000*	9.7 billion*
Medical care charges for small sample of AIDS patients in New York, Philadelphia, and San Francisco in 1984.[52]	56 weeks	168	1,003	168,000	45.4 billion

Description				
Medi-Cal expenditures for 1,103 AIDS patients from July 1983 to August 1986. Expenditures date from the onset of AIDS symptoms, which was often prior to actual AIDS diagnosis.[53]	78 weeks	NA	NA	77,000†	20.9 billion†
Medical care charges for 85 patients treated exclusively at San Francisco General Hospital who died in 1984.[54]	32 weeks	35	934	32,000	8.8 billion
Presents a range of charge estimates intended to be widely reflective of U.S. experience.[55]	NA	Low: 41 Medium: 63 High: 102	845† 971† 1,085†	43,000†‡ 68,000†‡ 115,000†‡	11.7 billion † 18.3 billion † 31.0 billion †
Medical costs for 45 patients with AIDS at New England Deaconess Hospital.[56]	NA	67	775*	55,000*†	14.9 billion*†

Source: D. E. Bloom, "The Economic Impact of AIDS in the United States," *Science* 239 (February 5, 1988): 604ff. Copyright © 1988 by the AAAS. Reprinted by permission of the author and publisher.
*Costs, as opposed to charges.
†Includes outpatient costs or charges.
‡These figures were estimated by using the detailed prevalence and cost figures reported in Scitovsky and Rice.[57]

APPENDIX B

Cumulative Savings Associated with Hospice Relative to Conventional Care Costs over the Last Year of Life

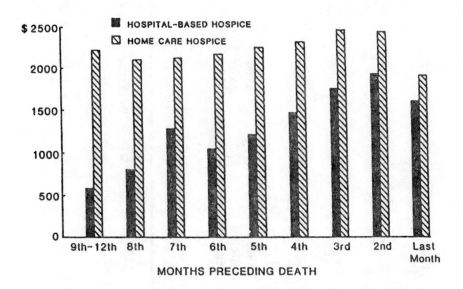

Source: V. Mor and D. Kidder, "Cost Savings in Hospice: Final Results of the National Hospice Study," *Health Services Research* 20, no. 4 (1985): 407–22. Reprinted with permission from the Hospital Research and Educational Trust.

NOTES

1. J. J. Johnson, *AIDS: An Overview of Issues* (CRS Report No. 1B87150) (Washington, D.C.: The Library of Congress, 1991).

2. M. Merlis, *Acquired Immune Deficiency Syndrome (AIDS): Health Care Financing and Services* (CRS Report No. 1B87219) (Washington, D.C.: The Library of Congress, 1990).

3. J. E. Sisk, "The Cost of AIDS: A Review of the Estimates," *Health Affairs* 6, no. 2 (1987): 5–20.

4. A. M. Hardy et al., "The Economic Impact of the First 10,000 Cases of Acquired Immunodeficiency Syndrome in the United States," *Journal of the American Medical Association* 255, no. 2 (1986): 19–31.

5. Institute of Medicine, "Care of Persons Infected with HIV," *Confronting AIDS, Update 1988* (Washington, D.C.: National Academy Press, 1988), pp. 93–121.

6. A. A. Scitovsky, "Studying the Cost of HIV-Related Illnesses: Reflections of a Moving Target," *The Millbank Quarterly* 67, no. 2 (1989): 318–46.

7. A. A. Scitovsky, M. Cline, and P. R. Lee, "Medical Care Costs of Patients with AIDS in San Francisco," *Journal of the American Medical Association* 256, no. 22: 3103–3106; G. R. Seage et al., "Medical Case Costs of AIDS in Massachusetts," *Journal of the American Medical Association* 256, no. 22 (1986): 3107–3109.

8. A. A. Scitovsky and D. P. Rice, "Estimates of the Direct and Indirect Costs of Acquired Immunodeficiency Syndrome in the United States, 1985, 1986, and 1991," *Public Health Reports* 102, no. 1 (1987): 5–17. For more detail on frequently cited studies of medical care costs for persons with AIDS, see Appendix A.

9. Ibid.

10. Ibid.

11. J. E. Sisk, "The Cost of AIDS: A Review of the Estimates," *Health Affairs* 6, no. 2 (1987): 5–20.

12. G. R. Seage et al., "Effect of Changing Patterns of Care and Duration of Survival on the Cost of Treating the Acquired Immunodeficiency Syndrome (AIDS)," *American Journal of Public Health* 80, no. 7 (1990): 835–39; Sisk, "The Cost of AIDS."

13. Sisk, "The Cost of AIDS."

14. Scitovsky, "Studying the Cost of HIV-Related Illnesses."

15. Sisk, "The Cost of AIDS."

16. Scitovsky, "Studying the Cost of HIV-Related Illnesses."

17. Institute of Medicine, "Care of Persons Infected with HIV."

18. J. K. Iglehart et al., "The Socioeconomic Impact of AIDS on Health Care Systems," *Health Affairs* 6, no. 3 (1987): 137–47.

19. P. S. Arno, "The Nonprofit Sector's Response to the AIDS Epidemic: Community-Based Services in San Francisco," *American Journal of Public Health* 76, no. 11 (1986): 1325–30.

20. Scitovsky, "Studying the Cost of HIV-Related Illnesses."

21. J. Green et al., "Projecting the Impact of AIDS on Hospitals," *Health Affairs* 6, no. 3 (1987): 19–31.

22. D. P. Andrulis et al., "The Provision and Financing of Medical Care for AIDS Patients in the U.S. Public and Private Teaching Hospitals," *Journal of the American Medical Association* 258, no. 10 (1987): 1343–46.

23. Institute of Medicine, "Care of Persons Infected with HIV."

24. W. L. Roper and W. Winkenwerder, "Making Fair Decisions about Financing Care for Persons with AIDS," *Public Health Reports* 103, no. 3: 305–308.

25. Merlis, *AIDS: Health Care Financing and Services.*

26. Ibid.; Sisk, "The Cost of AIDS."

27. L. Beresford, "Alternative Outpatient Settings of Care for People with AIDS," *Quarterly Review Bulletin* 1 (1989): 9–16.

28. P. A. Kawata and J. M. Andriote, "NAN–A National Voice for Community-Based Services for Persons with AIDS," *Public Health Reports* 103, no. 3 (1988): 299–304.

29. Scitovsky, Kline, and Lee, "Medical Care Costs of Patients with AIDS in San Francisco."

30. V. Mor and D. Kidder, "Cost Savings in Hospice: Final Results of the National Hospice Study," *Health Services Research* 20, no. 4 (1988): 407–22.

31. A. E. Benjamin, "Long-Term Care and AIDS: Perspectives from Experience with the Elderly," *The Milbank Quarterly* 66, no. 3 (1988): 415–43.

32. E. M. Howell, "The Role of Community-Based Organiza-

tions in Responding to the AIDS Epidemic: Examples from the HRSA Service Demonstration," *Journal of Public Health Policy* 12, no. 2 (1991): 165–73.

33. J. P. Martin, "Ensuring Quality Hospice Care for the Person with AIDS," *Quality Review Bulletin* 10 (1986): 353–58.

34. Beresford, "Alternative Outpatient Settings of Care for People with AIDS."

35. Benjamin, "Long-Term Care and AIDS."

36. S. J. Landers and G. R. Seage, "Medical Care of AIDS in New England: Costs and Implications," in P. O'Malley, ed., *The AIDS Epidemic: Private Rights and Public Interest* (Boston: Beacon Press, 1989), pp. 257–72.

37. Benjamin, "Long-Term Care and AIDS."

38. B. S. Bloom and P. D. Kissick, "Home and Hospital Cost of Terminal Illness," *Medical Care* 18, no. 5: 560–64.

39. Mor and Kidder, "Cost Savings in Hospice: Final Results of the National Hospice Study."

40. Arno, "The Nonprofit Sector's Response to the AIDS Epidemic."

41. Scitovsky, Kline, and Lee, "Medical Care Costs of Patients with AIDS in San Francisco."

42. In Landers and Seage, "Medical Care of AIDS in New England."

43. Beresford, "Alternative Outpatient: Settings of Care for People with AIDS."

44. Benjamin, "Long-Term Care and AIDS."

45. Beresford, "Alternative Outpatient Settings of Care for People with AIDS"; Benjamin, "Long-Term Care and AIDS."

46. Institute of Medicine, "Care of Persons Infected with HIV."

47. Merlis, *AIDS: Health Care Financing and Services.*

48. R. Rothenberg et al., "Survival with the Acquired Immunodeficiency Syndrome. Experience with 5,833 Cases in New York City," *The New England Journal of Medicine* 317, no. 21 (1987): 1297–1302.

49. K. W. Kizer et al., "An Updated Quantitative Analysis of AIDS in California," unpublished report of the California Department of Health Services, Sacramento.

50. Andrulis et al., "The Provision and Financing of Medical Care for AIDS Patients in U.S. Public and Private Teaching Hospitals," pp. 1343–46.

51. R. Berger, "Cost of AIDS Patients in Maryland," *Maryland State Medical Journal* 34 (1986): 1173.

52. Hardy et al., "The Economic Impact of the First 10,000 Cases of Acquired Immunodeficiency Syndrome in the United States," pp. 19–31.

53. Kizer et al., "Survival with the Acquired Immunodeficiency Syndrome," pp. 1297–1302.

54. Scitovsky et al., "Medical Care Costs of Patients with AIDS in San Francisco," pp. 3103–3106.

55. Scitovsky and Rice, "Estimates of the Direct and Indirect Costs of Acquired Immunodeficiency Syndrome in the United States, 1985, 1986, and 1991," pp. 5–17.

56. G. R. Seage et al. "Medical Care Costs of AIDS in Massachusetts," *Journal of the American Medical Association* 256, no. 22 (1986): 3107–3109.

57. Scitovsky and Rice, "Estimates of the Direct and Indirect Costs of Acquired Immunodeficiency Syndrome in the United States, 1985, 1986, and 1991," pp. 3103–3106.

8

Suicide, the Person with AIDS, and Hospice Care

The issue of suicide is one that the hospice team must be concerned with in their dealings with people with AIDS, their lovers, and families. Some people simply cannot deal with the complications and degeneration accompanying infection with HIV. Along with the proliferation of AIDS cases, the rate of suicide among people with AIDS is increasing at an alarming rate.

RATES OF SUICIDE AMONG PEOPLE WITH AIDS

The time when an individual with the AIDS virus is at risk of suicide has been defined as the duration of life. In a study of the rate of suicide among persons with AIDS in New York City for the year 1985, the person-years at risk of suicide were determined by the months at risk and then tabulated individually for males and females by quinary cohort, and then divided by twelve. The relative risk of suicide in an age and gender-specific AIDS cohort was calculated as the ratio of the suicide rate of the cohort to that of the general population. In New York City in 1985, there were 668 suicides, with the overall suicide rate being 18.75 deaths per one hundred thousand person-years of life. Of these 668 suicides, twelve were men aged twenty to fifty-nine who had been diagnosed with AIDS. This represents a rate of 680.56 deaths per one hundred thousand years of life for men with AIDS in this age group, which is 36.30 times that of men in this same age group not diagnosed with AIDS.[2] Of the twelve men who committed suicide, seven were white, three Hispanic, and two black; their average age was thirty-six. Nine of them were homosexual. All committed suicide within nine months of receiving their diagnosis of AIDS. The majority committed suicide within six months of diagnosis.[3]

Psychological reactions of persons with AIDS to the virus are common and vary with the individual patient. Due to societal pressure and condemnation, people with AIDS assume a burden of guilt for having brought the disease on themselves by their participation in such "taboo" activities as bisexuality, sex with multiple partners, or IV-drug use. When people with AIDS feel this way, they may look for forgiveness from others or else look for peace and solace through religion, hypnosis, or other methods. Patients who are not homosexual, bisexual, or IV-drug abusers feel particularly victimized by society, as may families and partners of people with AIDS.[4]

AIDS patients have often lost their lovers and are on their own. This gives them a feeling of being rejected or abandoned. Patients also have to deal with other losses, including dreams for the future, potential career and work-related goals, future travel plans, and satisfying human relationships. All these are factors goading the patient to commit suicide. Suicidal thoughts are also found in the lovers, spouses, and families of people with AIDS. The grieving process following an AIDS patient's death includes such severe depression factors as unrealistic guilt, helplessness, and loss of intimacy. Grief will be intensified if the lover or spouse has unknowingly infected his or her loved one. The climate surrounding AIDS is such that even those who think they have the virus might contemplate suicide.

The following case studies are illustrative:

Case Studies

A forty-year-old white homosexual male attempted suicide but was successfully resuscitated. The patient reported increased stress over the possibility that he had contracted AIDS; he refused testing because, he said, "it would only confirm the obvious." This man had a previous history of depression and attempted suicide, precipitated by the belief that he was already infected. The patient subsequently underwent therapy and medication; when he was tested for the AIDS virus, the results were negative. Six months later, he got involved in a support group for survivors of suicide attempts.[5]

A fifty-year-old black woman attempted suicide by overdosing with haloperidol (an antipsychotic drug) after her son died of AIDS. It was found that she had attempted suicide six months earlier because of a delusion that her terminally ill son was trying to kill her. The son spent the last few weeks of his life in a nursing home, with his mother by his side. There they formed a pact that they would die together. Since being put on medication to combat depression and undergoing counseling, the woman has suffered no recurrence of psychosis, suicidal behavior, or overt depression.[6]

A homosexual man with alcoholism and anxiety disorders contracted the AIDS virus after making several attempts on his life and having suicidal thoughts. He said that he wanted to die but had found it difficult to take his own life. The man was promiscuous and had put other people at risk of contracting the disease, because he slept with people already infected and individuals whose lovers had AIDS. This man would feel better about himself once alcohol had reduced the anxiety and distanced him from his problems; but he became depressed once more when the AIDS virus was diagnosed. However, he continued to reach out for help.[7]

These cases indicate that "suicide attempts related to AIDS are not confined to sufferers of the disease. Increasingly, people's fear of becoming infected or their despair over a loved one's death from the disease reaches suicidal proportions."[8] The ratio of female to male suicide attempts is about three to one; but the rate of actual suicides is three times higher for men. This could be because women suffer less psychiatric morbidity than usually appears in suicidal tendencies. Another reason could be that women have a much lower rate of alcohol abuse and dependency than men. "The interaction between HIV infection and suicidal ideation is complex and poorly understood."[9]

THE PSYCHIATRIC STATUS OF AIDS-RELATED SUICIDES*

The high rate of AIDS-related suicide is comparable to that of major psychiatric disorders. This suggests that biological mechanisms might be contributory factors. AIDS is strongly associated with psychiatric syndromes, including depression, psychosis, and dementia.[10] Intravenous drug abusers, for example, are at a high risk of suicide because they are in such a state of depression. Psychiatric disorders provide a profile of how psychopathology may contribute to the cause and course of AIDS. There is much need for more research into this area.

Organic brain syndromes associated with AIDS are frequently undiagnosed or misdiagnosed. Sometimes they are associated with neurologic findings and sometimes not. *Delirium* is found very often in patients with AIDS. The individual's level of awareness is reduced and thinking, perceiving, and remembering are all impaired. *Dementia* involves a loss of intellectual abilities and can affect the individual's social and occupational functioning. *Organic mood disorder* occurs where there is an organic cause of disturbance, with a depressive or manic episode. Major depression can result in insomnia or hypersomnia and psychomotor retardation or agitation, and it is characterized by depressed mood, guilt, loss of interest, and hopelessness. It may also involve suicidal thoughts.[11] *Organic delusions* seem to be paranoid and grandiose; for example, one may believe oneself to be Jesus Christ.

---

*For a list of organic and other disorders, see the appendix at the end of this chapter.

THE ROLE OF HOSPICE IN ASSISTING THE ILL AND DYING

Counseling

A psychosocial questionnaire distributed to AIDS victims asked the respondents how their careers had been affected by the illness and whether it had changed their social relationships. Patients replied that their sexuality had diminished, the reasons being reduced energy and libido, fear of transmitting AIDS through sexual contact, and markedly decreased frequency of social contacts. There were several patients who said that they developed or maintained intimate relationships that were not dependent on sexual expression. Others replied that they had reduced frequency of social interactions with friends. All respondents said that they wanted more educational support, more emotional support, more of a sense that society was making every effort to combat AIDS, and a comprehensive treatment program that attended to their medical and psychosocial needs.[12]

When the infected individual finally gets past the denial stage, then the "Why me?" syndrome may occur. Eventually, people with AIDS will break down and face reality as well as deal with the problems created by the illness. Patients can be bolstered psychologically by the treatment and assistive support they receive, but frequently the psychological impact of the illness is so devastating that anxiety, denial, anger, depression, and suicidal thoughts predominate.

Anxiety may be defined as "the 'unpleasure' experienced by the individual when the anticipation of being overwhelmed by an internal and external force is present." Patients who have just been diagnosed with AIDS can experience an intense anxiety reaction. Although anxiety is a normal reaction to a life-threatening illness, patients sometimes face continuous generalized anxiety, phobias, and even panic attacks. Fear might cause the patient to become demanding or dependent and mistrusting of the hospice care team. "The overall goal of intervention with anxious persons with AIDS is to assist them to accept the illness and regain the ability to manage their lives."[13]

A psychiatric nurse helps deal with the HIV epidemic both by providing pretest counseling that considers the needs of the individual and encompassing the sensitivity and prognostic meaning of the test;

medical history; and assessment of risk factors, vulnerabilities, coping capacities, and supportive resources. "Findings indicate that pretest and post-test counseling can provide an opportunity to identify a subpopulation at risk for psychiatric morbidity."[14]

Suicide Prevention

The question of assisted suicide or active euthanasia is one of very serious concern to physicians. The attitudes of society toward the terminally ill, including individual autonomy and the physician's role, are not easily dismissed. Given hospice's emphasis on palliative rather than aggressive medical or resuscitative procedures, it possibly risks the charge that it's killing, not helping, patients. "Only caring for the terminally ill patients, rather than subjecting them to inappropriate treatments that only prolong the process of dying, is quite different, both clinically and morally, from assisted suicide or active euthanasia. . . . Although the illness is terminal, efforts at suicide prevention are appropriate to allow patients to rationally evaluate alternatives to treatment, to integrate their lives in terms of financial and other planning, and to allow resolution of personal relationships with family and friends."[15]

Care for AIDS patients with suicidal thoughts is a very serious matter and should never be taken as a joke. Care providers must look for certain signs; for example, the inability to concentrate and difficulty in making decisions can indicate that an individual is thinking of suicide. Diagnosing depression is not always easy—small things like weight loss, change in sleep patterns, fatigue, and changes in activity levels are all signs of depression. Once the staff discovers that a patient is depressed, they should try gradually to draw out his or her feelings, basically leading up to the question, "Are things so bad that you are thinking of suicide?" If the patient says yes, the staff should immediately consider the situation an emergency, and check to see if there any weapons or pills around and whether the patient has any specific plans for them. The main thing to remember is to ask about suicide "by including [patients] in all possible decisions, providing them with the information they need for decision making, and helping them explore their options."[16]

When dealing with patients who are hopelessly ill, however, the matter of resuscitation comes up. Since the technique of cardiopulmonary resuscitation has been improved, the question of when to use it has arisen. Sometimes an instruction can be put on the patient's order sheet stating that there should be no resuscitation; it must be signed by a doctor. New organizations, like Dying with Dignity and the Society for the Right to Die, advocate the use of a document that permits individuals to request in advance not to be resuscitated or kept alive by artificial means. This document is called the living will. The taking of their own life by the terminally ill might eventually be viewed as a rational and acceptable act under certain conditions; this, however, conflicts with the current psychiatric viewpoint that to attempt suicide is a manifestation of mental illness.[17]

Consider "Mr. B," a middle-aged homosexual suffering from AIDS, who underwent a mood swing following a negative change in his condition. After being released from the hospital, he was admitted to a medical ward two weeks later due to an overdose of sleeping medication. He was let go due to his improved mood, only to be readmitted one week later because of increasing weakness. Mr. B's condition deteriorated to such a point that a "do not resuscitate" order was placed on his chart. Four weeks later he was found in a comatose state with an empty vial of an unprescribed medication next to him. Resuscitative measures were not taken and he died.

In another case, an individual made a living will and gave it to his children. Three years later, the children found him unconscious due to a suspected overdose; they rushed him to a hospital, where emergency-room physicians successfully resuscitated him, even though family members insisted that these efforts were contrary to their father's wishes. The man was in good physical and emotional health prior to the attempted suicide, but he still considers his act a thoughtful and rational one.[18]

"It has not been established in American law whether withholding resuscitation in these circumstances is distinct from the act of suicide. Further discussion and research into this most difficult area would be welcome. Ultimately, the appropriate response in cases such as those presented must be formulated on the basis of an amalgam of patients' rights and wishes, physicians' rights and responsibilities, and the legal imperatives."[19]

Other Considerations

The way a physician or a nurse feels about a patient often weighs heavily in determining the quality of medical care. Positive regard for a patient has long been among the most powerful therapeutic tools. However, caring for the patient with AIDS can be very deadly if the individual does not follow certain precautions. A handful of health professionals have been infected with the AIDS virus through casual contact with blood. Therefore, health care workers may regard every AIDS patient as a potential enemy. According to a recent survey, more than 25 percent of young physicians would not take care of AIDS patients if they were given the choice. "This dreadful disease is not only killing young people in the prime of life and destroying their familial and social relationships, it also is damaging the bond between the caregiver and the patient with AIDS as well."[20]

People with AIDS suffer in so many different ways. Each is faced with severe illnesses, weight loss, weakness, fevers, disfigurements, blindness, and psychiatric disorders. It is the care provider's objective to keep patients' spirits up through all of these problems. Cognitive approval of the crisis is crucial for the patient.

Many patients have indicated that spirituality is important to them. However, spirituality has been avoided by professional caregivers because they choose to put their emphasis on other components of care. They stay clear of it because they feel they are unqualified. Hence the choice of spiritual guidance may be left to the individual hospice care program.

CONCLUSION

Overall, hospice is very successful in relieving the suicidal thoughts in AIDS patients that may arise due to intractable pain, physical degeneration, and feelings of hopelessness and despair. At the same time, it recognizes that it is helping patients along the road to death.

The concept of hospice is based on the dying words of Mark Twain, "No ship can outsail death. . . . When I seem to be dying, I do not want to be stimulated back to life." The hospice team works with families and patients, providing constant companionship, reassurance, and pain and symptom control. Hospice has learned how to change the common causes of death. In a death-denying society, it helps provide a loving and caring environment where patients may live out their remaining days in a positive atmosphere. The affirmative concept of hospice is spelled out in the following statement of the National Hospice Organization: Hospice affirms life, recognizing that dying is a normal process, which hospice neither hastens nor postpones.

NOTES

1. Clark et al., "Hospice Care: A Model for Caring for the Person with AIDS," *Nurses Clin. North America* 23, no. 4 (December 1988): 851–62.

2. Elizabeth Carr, "Psychosocial Issues of AIDS Patients in Hospice: Case Studies," *The Hospice Journal* (1989): 143.

3. Marzuk et al., "Increased Risk of Suicide in Persons with AIDS," *Journal of the American Medical Association* (March 4, 1988): 29.

4. Mary Cohen, "Biopsychosocial Approach to the Human Immunodeficiency Virus Epidemic," *General Hospital Psychiatry* (1990): 110–112.

5. Karlinsky et al., "Suicide Attempts and Resuscitation Dilemmas," *General Hospital Psychiatry* (1988): 423.

6. Ibid., p. 424.

7. Steven Lippmann Frierson, "Suicide and AIDS," *Psychosomatics* (Spring 1988): 228.

8. Karlinsky, et al., "Suicide Attempts and Resuscitation Dilemmas," p. 425.

9. Frances et al., "Contracting AIDS as a Means of Committing Suicide," *American Journal of Psychiatry* (May 1985): 142.

10. Donlon et al., "Psychosocial Aspects of AIDS and AIDS-

Related Complex: A Pilot Study," *Journal of Psychosocial Oncology* (Summer 1985): 48–51.

11. Ibid., pp. 46–47

12. Perry et al., "Suicidal Ideation and HIV Testing," *Journal of the American Medical Association* (February 2, 1990): 679–82.

13. Saunders, and Stephan Buckingham, "When the Depression Turns Deadly," *Nursing* (July 1988): 62.

14. David Rogers, "Caring for the Patient with AIDS," *Journal of the American Medical Association* (March 1988): 1368.

15. Cohen, "Biopsychological Approach to the Human Immunodeficiency Virus Epidemic," p. 98.

16. Millison, and James Dudley, "The Importance of Spirituality in Hospice Work: A Study of Hospice Professionals," *Hospice Journal* (1990): 67–69.

17. Marzuk et al., "The Risk of Suicide in Persons with AIDS," *Journal of the American Medical Association* (July 1, 1988): 1334

18. Carr, "Psychosocial Issues of AIDS Patients in Hospice: Case Studies," p. 142.

19. Ibid.

20. Zerwekh, and Ann Blues, "Hospice and Palliative Nursing Care," *Journal of Psychosocial Oncology*: 113–114.

APPENDIX

Psychiatric Disorders Associated with HIV Infection*

Organic mental disorders:

Dementia

HIV dementia or AIDS-dementia complex

Dementia associated with opportunistic infections and cancers

Infections

Fungal

Cryptococcoma

Cryptococcal meningitis

Candida abscesses

Protozoal

Toxoplasmosis

Bacterial

Mycobacterium avium intracellulare (MAI)

Viral

Cytomegalovirus

Herpes virus

Papovavirus progressive multifocal

Leukoencephalopathy

Cancers

---

*Adapted from Gwen van Servellen Nyamanthi, "Maladaptive Coping in the Critically Ill Population with Acquired Immunodeficiency Syndrome: Nursing Assessment and Treatment," *Heart and Lung* (March 1989): 115–16.

Primary cerebral lymphoma

Disseminated Kaposi's sarcoma

Delirium:

Organic delusional disorder

Organic mood disorder

Depressed

Manic

Mixed

Affective disorders

Major depression

Dysthymic disorder

Adjustment disorders

Adjustment disorder with depressed mood

Adjustment disorder with anxious mood

Substance abuse disorder

Borderline personality disorder

Antisocial personality disorder

Epilogue

A Chorus of Friends
Ralph O. Hall

JEANETTE'S FAMILY VERSUS AIDS

AIDS is a deadly killer. Evidence is available in a January 1990 obituary notice of the *Mankato Free Press*.

> Donnie Gimmer, 24, died after a prolonged illness. He is survived by family members: daughter, Cassie, and her mother, Gina; father, Les, and mother, Jeanette; sisters, Midge, Deb, and Shari; brothers, Ralph, Lawrence, and Les; numerous nieces and nephews. He was preceded in death by his brother Charlie in 1981 at age 33.

Any family engaged in the battle to survive the conflict caused by this disease is presently facing certain tragedy. There is only a glimmer of hope coming from the medical researchers. Any hope of successfully surviving the ordeal of AIDS today will be found in the strength of the family engaged in the battle, and reinforced with the compassion and care of the invaluable hospice caregiver.

This story of Jeanette's family is told through the voices of suffering family members. These voices are presented in a choral manner,
first combined in these introductory paragraphs, separated and indi-
vidualized in the body of the epilogue, and combined again in the
acknowledgments at the end. It is the combination of voices that
will provide the ultimate weapon against the enemy, AIDS.

Acquired Immunodeficiency Syndrome crashed on the world less
than one decade before Donnie's death in 1990. By crashed, we mean
claimed victims next door or made the news on the local television
station. Public health information, supported by various national
religious ministries, early on pointed to homosexual relationships or
drug use as the likely means of transmission of this virus that was
claiming victims at an epidemic rate worldwide. Our family was not
willing to announce the real cause of Donnie's death, thereby putting
another burden on his tortured soul, and, with that, casting an
additional shadow on our own lives.

AIDS is a frightening companion, presently bringing with it feelings of hopelessness in the discovery of the medical cure, embarrass-
ment over the class of society labeled as high-risk, pity for the agoniz-
ingly long and lonely deterioration of the body of the afflicted, and
fear of the still unknown transmission and incubation patterns of
the virus. A person who contracts this affliction is headed down
a dark road indeed. The strength to hold one's head up during the
trek is difficult to acquire and even more difficult to maintain. The
hospice care we have received has helped us to keep our strength up.

Before you can truly hear our individual voices, a few facts and
general characteristics need to be presented as background. We hope
you find these helpful in setting the stage for the chorus of family members who make up this story.

We feel that AIDS is only the current chapter in the story of
a family already burdened with the hereditary blood disorder known
as hemophilia. This disease is relatively uncommon, with only about
100,000 known cases in the Western world. It might even be more
unknown were it not for the existence of this condition in Queen
Victoria's consort, Albert, and their offspring. Her issue, successfully
dowered to the other regal households, "carried" the deadly gene
to the royal families of the European continent. Hence hemophilia

earned the nickname "royal disease." Most notable was Princess Alexandra of Germany, who married Czar Nicholas of Russia. Their son's hemophilia is a story affecting world history, one well told by Robert Massie in his *Nicholas and Alexandra.*

Hemophilia is an inability of the blood to clot. There are ten "factorates" that cause blood to coagulate when exposed to conditions outside the blood vessels; the absence of one or more of these factorates results in continuous bleeding beyond normal time limits. Such external bleeding can lead to death. Internal bleeding leads to much discomfort at such sites as joints or pouches.* A residue of blood can lead to an arthritic-like restriction of use.

One of the more vital factorates of this clotting process carries the label "factor eight," the instructions for whose "manufacture" are missing from our family's genetic transmission. The statistical probability of inheriting the inability to manufacture factor eight is exactly 50 percent. This genetic pattern is transmitted by the X chromosome. The Mendelian genetic flow chart for three generations looks like this:

XX = female, XY = male, x = missing factor 8, I = the connector

```
                          xX          XY
                        carrier     normal

            XX          XY          xX          xY
          normal      normal      carrier     bleeder
                                     I           I
                                     I           I
            XX XY       xX          xY  I
          normal      carrier     bleeder        I
                                                 I
                                     I
                                   XY XY       xX xX
                                  normal      carrier
```

---

*Internal pools of blood in the back, breast, and stomach cavities

The mother is labeled a "carrier" because the existence of a second X chromosome brings with it the ability to produce factor eight; hence she does not suffer bleeds but can pass the gene on. The male Y chromosome does not have that ability, but the deficient trait was seldom passed on due to a high mortality rate among males. Modern-day medicine has changed this pattern so that males live into their child-begetting years and they, too, have become carriers.

The medical evolution of a cure for hemophilia has taken more than 150 years. The study of genetics led to an understanding of its transmission, which led in turn to the discovery of the ten factors essential to clotting. The exploration of the nature of blood has presented the medical profession with a progression of treatments for the missing factor(s). Up to the 1950s, whole blood transfusions were administered until the clotting could take place naturally or through replacement of factor-deficient blood. Increased knowledge of the clotting process has led to a refinement of knowledge about how the blood components parcel out a substance known as cryo-precipitate (cryo), and finally to the slippery factorate itself. With this substance administered on a periodic basis, and care taken to avoid injurious situations, the prospect of living as normal a life as a diabetic had arrived. Hemophiliacs needed to concern themselves now with education, job training, and even family preparation. Like many other afflicted families, Jeanette and her eight children were assimilating themselves into the mainstream.

That assimilation came to an abrupt end in 1981. Jeanette's oldest son, Charles, ended a life of suffering and avoided a bleak future by pulling the trigger of a rifle whose muzzle was carefully inserted in his mouth. AIDS was not discussed as a component of the answer to the tearful question "Why?" Lifelong pain from the bleeds, immobility of the joints, unsuccessful knee-replacement operations, addiction to relief-supplying drugs, and a future of impending helplessness were answer enough at the time. AIDS was unknown to our family in 1981. In the ten years since then, we have been engaged in a death-grip struggle with the disease that has made itself horribly well known. We do not know whether Charlie had knowledge of the looming disaster of AIDS.

The stories began quietly enough in the pages of medical journals and progressed to the general news. A new strain of virus that attacked the human immune system was amassing victims at an alarming rate. Its origins lay apparently in Africa and it was transmitted primarily through commingling of human body fluids. People who shared body fluids, initially identified as homosexual males and needle-using drug addicts, later became known as "high risk groups."

AIDS made the front pages of American newspapers with the death of actor Rock Hudson in 1985. But there is a high-risk group not publicized in the media, who receive medical supervision and pay dearly for that treatment and care. The nation's hemophiliacs number about 25,000, of whom 70 percent are testing positive for HIV. Hemophiliacs are considered among the highest risk groups. The very blood products recommended to alleviate the affliction had introduced us to AIDS.

In our family group, all three of the remaining bleeders are afflicted with the virus. Lawrence, fondly known as Scott, endures a fluctuating white blood and T-cell count indicative of ongoing immune system depresssion. Les endures constant fatigue, weight and appetite loss, and nuisance infections. Both are presently making plans to face death. Donnie passed away in 1990 from AIDS-Related Complex (ARC).

Our family is facing this both as a group and separately. On the one hand, the adversity draws us together as a clan to elicit the strength of all when the individual falters. On the other hand, we each face our individual agony depending on the aspect of AIDS that presents itself. Our separate families have still another perspective on this ongoing battle.

Chester Kersting and Irma Widgery had one child, a daughter, Jeanette. Jeanette has been married three times in her life, giving birth to eight children.

Midge, named Irma after her grandmother, was the first born. She has two daughters, Jody and Julie, who each have children of their own.

Charles, the most severe of the bleeders, fathered one son, Allan, before his death.

Ralph, forty-two, is the only son of five to not be afflicted as a bleeder. He has three children, Jenny, Kelley, and Alex, and is presently married to Sharon Kay.

Lawrence, thirty-nine, attained important family firsts: a bacca-laureate degree, master's degree, and a doctorate. He has chosen to remain a bachelor.

Les, thirty-seven, married Val in 1985. Their family includes Melanie, Amber, and Melina. Our family's attention is presently focused on the battle against his serious illness.

Debbie, thirty-five and married to Blaine, is the only known carrier among the daughters. Her son, Shaundelle, is the only grandson afflicted with bleeds. She has a daughter, Heidie.

Sharon—or Shari—thirty-two, is married to Steve. They have two children, Matt and Sara, who do not exhibit any signs of hemophilia.

Donnie would now be nearly twenty-six had he not been the first to succumb in the battle against AIDS. He and Gina made Jeanette a grandma for the eleventh time with Cassie.

Our distribution of the hemophilia gene is outside probability. Four of the five sons are bleeders and one of three daughters is a known carrier (the two others are unsure at this time). The next generation is more fortunate. Of the eleven grandchildren, only one is a bleeder and two are carriers.

By combining our family strength, increasing public awareness that the battle is in the mainstream of life, and gathering the forces of hospice support now beginning to emerge, we will not only survive these battles, but we will win the war. The perceptions that follow are from family members who want to say how they feel. From this collection of voices, you can, at once, hear the bonding that adversity offers and the divergence that longing for freedom from suffering brings. Here are their individual voices.

GINA AND CASSIE

I am the mother of Donnie Gimmer's daughter, Cassandra Gimmer.

Watch someone you love die and then try to explain that to a three-year-old. Her daddy is sick and dying. She asks "Why?" It is really hard to watch someone you love totally change. From loving, tall, and fun to be with—then change to weight loss, sleep a lot, begin to look old and suffer so much, not to be able to eat, mouth so sore, and not even able to remember your own little girl. I, still to this day, love Donnie and so does Cassie. I never want her to forget him. She is now five-and-a-half-years-old and I know someday soon I will have to explain it to her all over again.

After Donnie died, Cassie and I cried for two days. It was hard for me. I spent seven years of my life with him.

Now we go out to the cemetery on all holidays, birthdays, Father's Day, or whenever we need to. When we just drive by, we honk and wave and tell him we still love him.

SHARON K. HALL

The majority of my feelings and reactions to this family's battle, first with hemophilia, and now AIDS, are directly related to the effect these two diseases have had on Ralph's life.

I had known Ralph only a few months when his older brother, Charlie, took his life. It appeared that hemophilia (and its results) had taken its toll on Charlie's ability to live life as he would have chosen. Consequently, in 1981, Charlie ended his own life. I believe that this was not a selfish act, nor an act of cowardice. Charlie had endured years of pain and some degree of humiliation, because he doggedly struggled to achieve the same physical activities as "normal" males.

With Charlie's death came my first insight into the strength and closeness of the family. I was amazed by the way they seemed to band together even closer to give each other strength and reassurance. It was at this time that Ralph became the "oldest son." He took charge of helping his bereaved mother make funeral arrangements and ended the funeral service by giving one of the most beautiful eulogies I've ever heard. I remember listening to Ralph speaking of his deceased older brother to the church full of mourners and thinking to myself, "I would never be able to do what he's doing. I'm just not strong enough!" I knew then that Ralph was a special human being.

As time went on and my friendship with Ralph grew, he shared his family's background with me. It was a medical background almost too unreal to be true. Unfortunately, only one brother out of five was not a bleeder. Grateful as I am that Ralph was spared hemophilia, I understand that he has nonetheless suffered along with his frail half-brothers.

He was naturally delegated the tasks that were too physically demanding (therefore, potentially dangerous) for his brothers to undertake. Ralph did this willingly and still had time and room to feel compassion for his brothers and mother. (I don't know if any resentment ever surfaced or was felt.) I do believe that Ralph felt a degree of guilt because he was his mother's only healthy son. I look on this as the reverse of when a person has just been informed that he or she has a dreaded disease and the first reaction is "Why me?"

As months turned into years, Ralph and I married. I saw Ralph's role as "big brother" become a way of life for him. I soon realized that his family looked up to him and depended on him. Even though Charlie's death was the first time I'd witnessed Ralph as the "big brother," I'm convinced this was the role he's always played in his family.

As if helplessly watching his brothers suffer hemophilia as children and then adults wasn't enough, Ralph was to be told that his youngest brother, Donnie, had tested positive for the AIDS virus. Donnie's diagnosis prompted the remaining two brothers to go for an HIV test as well. When their results were also positive, we concluded that the blood transfusions administered to all three brothers to combat the hemophilia had been tainted with the HIV virus. How ironic! The very method used to ease their bleeding and pain meant almost certain death.

Donnie was the first to die from AIDS complications. He passed away January 10, 1990, at the age of twenty-four. It was sad to see such a young man die. He left behind a three-year-old daughter who still misses him. Jeanette took Donnie's death terribly hard. She cared for him in her home right up to his death. Near the end, a local hospice group came to her assistance, allowing her to be relieved of the constant attendance at Donnie's side. I remember thinking, "How courageous the Prairie River Care Providers are." With the uncertainties surrounding transmission of the AIDS virus, it took courage as well as compassion to give Donnie this care.

Ralph wasn't close to Donnie. This was partly because of the sixteen-year age difference. In addition, Ralph and Donnie disagreed on the lifestyle chosen by Donnie. Donnie lived life in "the fast lane" and took risks that got him into trouble with the law as well as contributing to a more rapid deterioration due to AIDS.

Rapid deterioration from HIV complications include weight loss, physical fatigue, and a loss of appetite. Les, presently thirty-seven, is exhibiting these symptoms at an accelerating pace. Because we've all witnessed these signs as recently as 1990, we are fearful that Les won't be with us long. I am personally closer to Les than the other brothers, so I am experiencing a deeper sense of sadness and loss already.

I try to be here for Ralph when he feels like talking about it or when he wants to go visit with Les. As I have said, Ralph is a very strong person; but he may need someone to lean on now and again, and I want to be here when that need arises.

Scott is the brother two years younger than Ralph. His illness is not as advanced as Les's condition. Scott manages to maintain a strong, positive attitude. It doesn't matter if the attitude is only on the outside; it seems to help Scott and that helps the family members when they are around him.

We are all going through a sad and difficult time. It's so frustrating to know this is going to happen and you're helpless to stop it. I know that I speak for the entire family when I say, "I wish we'd never heard of HIV." The reality is—we have it, it's here, and we all have to learn to live (and die) with it.

I'm counting on Ralph to give them all the strength that he has given me. I was a victim of cancer several years ago. It was also a scary and sad experience. I remember the fear and the feelings of weakness and defenselessness. I came through that cursed disease and have been pronounced cured. I was lucky, there is a treatment and surgery for cancer. Presently there is no cure for AIDS. A significant contributing factor in my beating cancer was our sharing of strength. Each morning, Ralph would come to hug me and ask, "Do you feel the strength flowing into you?" You know what? I did. If only Ralph's hugs would return to Les and Scott their strength as well.

VAL

When Les and I first met in January 1978, our relationship was "insignificant." We were simply co-workers at the Regional Treatment Center in St. Peter, Minnesota. We worked with clients who are mentally retarded. At times, it was necessary for staff to intervene when clients became aggressive. At that time, I was not aware of Les's hemophilia, but I was impressed with his willingness to assist other staff with aggressive clients as the need arose. A few weeks after we began working together, Les responded to a call from another area of the hospital: staff were requesting help with a client who was acting up. Les's usual propensity to assist others resulted in a significant injury to his ankle. He was admitted to the hospital, where he was treated for a broken ankle and the bleeding that occurred in the tissues surrounding the fracture. Released after a ten-day hospitalization, Les was, however, unable to work for a few months while his ankle healed. Following the injury, he was frequently referred to as "Gimp" by friends and co-workers. The experience had left him with a permanent injury that periodically caused him to limp.

Later, I learned that the injury necessitated very large quantities of factorate, the blood product that allows the blood to clot. After the ankle injury, Les used factorate to treat less severe bleeds (in his elbow) on one or two more occasions. Early in 1982, Les first read about AIDS in a newspaper. After that, he refused to use blood products, choosing instead to treat the bleeds with ice and rest. At that time the medical profession continued to advise hemophilia patients to use blood products to assist in preventing arthritic conditions that invariably occurred as a result of untreated bleeds.

In 1983, Les and I became close friends. He was supportive of me through a very stressful time in my life. I found I could talk to him about anything. Several months after my marriage ended, we began dating and our relationship quickly became very close. In June of 1985, we were married. Les had taken on the responsibility of becoming a full-time parent to my daughters, Amber (then five) and Melina (then three). Les's daughter, Melanie (then nine) continued to live with her mother but periodically visited us with her sister, Patty (then eight).

Though Les talked about HIV and its relationship to hemophilia, it seemed as if the possibility that this horrible disease could touch us was remote. In 1985, the news media had begun to talk about AIDS more and more often, increasing my awareness of the disease. I was also learning more about hemophilia and its treatment, thus enabling me to understand the connection between the two diseases. Still, it seemed that Les had protected himself sufficiently by not using factorate for almost four years.

A few months after we were married, Les became ill with flu and cold symptoms. One of the lymph nodes in his neck became quite swollen and he had a chronic sore throat. These symptoms persisted and Les's concern that this could be related to AIDS increased. We went to the Mayo Clinic in Rochester, Minnesota, for guidance.

The doctors at Mayo reluctantly spoke with us about the possibility of Les being HIV-positive. Though it was estimated that 80 percent to 90 percent of hemophilia patients had been exposed to the virus, Les was advised *against* being tested. If he'd been exposed, there was little the doctors could do. Les insisted on being tested and the doctors finally agreed. We all felt that chances for testing negative would be greatly enhanced because he had not used factorate for almost four years. The test was performed in hopes of alleviating the stress of the unknown.

I'll never forget the day we were notified that the test was positive for HIV. We'd only been married for a few months and our life together was just getting started. Up to that point, I'd been at a stage of total denial that this could ever happen. Now we were faced with such questions as "How do we protect the children?" and "Who were Les's previous sexual contacts?" Though these issues seem quite trivial now, at the time they caused a great deal of pain. Horror stories about families in our same situation filled the news. We were fearful of being "shunned" by friends and co-workers. That night, Amber was to have a neighbor girl spend the night. Would her parents allow this if they knew?

For the first few months, we lived in a degree of secrecy. Initially, we informed only our families. Gradually, we were able to tell our closest friends and finally our co-workers without experiencing hostile reactions. Perhaps this was due to the fact that we both worked in a hospital setting where people are more medically knowledgeable. The fact that people have been so supportive and accepting of us has allowed us to "keep it together" to some extent over the past six years. These people may never know how thankful we are for their caring and accepting attitude.

In many ways, the first year was the most stresssful for Les. After finding out that he was infected, we had to deal with the fact that the doctors knew very little about the disease. We were told that Les's swollen lymph node, which continued to enlarge, was a result of his smoking. Then the doctors decided that the problem was probably a result of Les worrying over it. If he'd quit touching it so much, the swelling might go down! The sore throat, which continued to worsen, was also assumed to be a result of smoking, and the white coating Les found on his tongue was determined to be "nothing." His lack of energy was blamed on "depression," and Les was referred to a psychiatrist. Les was treated as someone who was overreacting to the symptoms now commonly associated with the virus.

Finally, the doctors decided to do a biopsy on the swollen lymph node. Les was admitted to the hospital in Rochester, where he was given factorate and the lymph node was removed. The doctors originally planned to release him from the hospital the same day, but decided to keep him for observation overnight to ensure that the bleeding in his neck had stopped. This entire experience was one of the worst we'd had.

Some of the nurses and interns came into the room with gowns and rubber gloves and still appeared to be fearful of going near Les. One particular staff person stands out. She entered the room with her gown and gloves and stood a full foot from the bed talking to him. Not once did this person touch Les, and it was obvious she was uncomfortable being in the same room with one infected with HIV.

The day after the surgery, Les was released from the hospital. By this time, he was extremely irritable and tense. He was worried that his clotting factor had not been retested to ensure that the postoperative bleeding in his neck would stop. For a day and a half, he'd been treated as a "leper" and each and every concern Les had was attributed to his "overreaction" to the disease. By the time of his release, Les was responding to this treatment by truly appearing as if he were neurotic. The doctor suggested "inpatient treatment" for his apparent "emotional problems." He was sent home with the understanding that he need not worry about his incision. The bleeding had stopped.

The tension in the car during the two-hour drive home was unbelievable. Still knowing little about AIDS and having blind trust in the medical profession, I attempted to treat Les's concerns as if he were truly overreacting. A few hours after we'd arrived home, I had to drive Les to the local hospital at Mankato. His airway was beginning to close from the bleeding and swelling around the incision in his neck. Les was hospitalized in Mankato for an additional week. He received factorate each day and excellent care.

After this experience, Les began to go to the HIV clinic at the University of Minnesota Hospital in Minneapolis. Our insurance provided better coverage there and we hoped that the existence of a large gay community in Minneapolis would have forced that hospital to keep abreast of the latest developments. Following his first visit, Les discovered that the sore throat he'd had for the past year, previously attributed to smoking, was in fact candidiasis, the yeast infection that commonly affects AIDS patients. Within a few days, Les began to respond to treatment. We also learned that his swollen lymph nodes were a result of the virus. Later, we were informed that the unexplained lack of energy was symptomatic of HIV infection.

Over the next few years, we attempted to live as normal a life as possible. In the summer of 1987, we hired a contractor to build a house, knowing that such a move could put us in financial stress later, if Les's condition worsened. As completion of the house was nearing, Les returned from a medical appointment with disturbing news: he'd been diagnosed with AIDS-Related Complex (ARC). Though we'd both been aware that many of his symptoms were related to the virus, being diagnosed with ARC suggested that the eventual onset of full-blown AIDS was not just possible but probable. After moving into the new house, Les began to feel better. For a period of time, he avoided going to the clinic, as each visit was proving to be stressful and it seemed as if nothing was being gained from them.

As time went on, the medical profession began to learn more and more about the disease process and how to monitor its progression through blood tests. When Les finally returned to the clinic, blood tests showed that his disease was progressing. He began to investigate various treatment options. There were only a few and all involved entering studies being performed on various drugs.

The most widely recognized treatment was AZT, but Les was unable to tolerate this new drug, which made him vomit with each trial. Determined to do what he could, he entered other drug study at the University of Minnesota and the Centers for Disease Control at Bethesda Hospital. Though each study involved a great deal of time, effort, periodic hospitalization, and frequent blood tests, the disease continued to progress. Les's T-4 count, one of the measurements used to evaluate the immune system's deterioration, had dropped from 500 (one-half the normal level) to 50 in less than three years.

Finally, Les began to receive (and was able to tolerate) DDI, a drug that held great promise. He has continued to receive this medication for eighteen months in an effort to slow the progression of the disease. At the present time, Les's condition is much worse. Though he continues to receive DDI and a number of other medications to deal with and/or prevent AIDS-related diseases and symptoms, the days that he awakens feeling well are nonexistent. On a "good" day, Les can eat without vomiting or maybe the neuropathy that causes chronic pain in his hands and feet subsides to the extent that he is able to drive a few miles.

Through the years, my coping mechanism has been denial. First, I was able to deny that Les had been infected. Then I was able to deny that being infected was necessarily a death sentence. I believed that something would be developed to effectively treat AIDS patients. My ability to deny has deteriorated along with Les's health, leaving me with a feeling of ambivalence. If I accept the idea of Les's death, will this attitude hasten his death? On the other hand, if I do not accept the fact that he will die, does this leave him alone to deal with death? Should the children be prepared for this now or wait?

Recently, Les completed a living will outlining the procedures he would and would not accept in the event he is incapable of decision making later. Though we readily agree on most portions of this document, Les surprised me by listing the hospital where he would want to die. Given the fact that he had always hated the hospital, I'd assumed that he would be at home at the time of his death. As is typical, Les explained that he thought this would be easier on the rest of the family. After some discussion he agreed to change this. When someone you love is dying of AIDS, there is little a person can do to make their life easier or to make them happy. To be there for someone you love, when they need you, is about all you can do. I pray that, if the time comes, I am there for Les. It is all I have to offer him. It is about all I can do.

SHARI
(IN MEMORY OF CHARLIE AND DONNIE)

My name is Sharon. I'm one of the eight children in this family who is trying to understand and accept the harsh realities of life. My family is living with AIDS.

The biggest questions are, "Why us, God? Why our family? And why three out of five of my brothers?" I know these are the sorts of questions that each of us asks at one time or another, for their own particular reasons or tragedies.

Everyone loves their family, just like I love my family. But when you have to stand back, helpless, your heart aches to do something. But what? Give them all the love and support you can. Be there for them, even when they reject you.

The feelings I always kept locked inside me, in a safe place, I can't help but let flow out of me, to extremes at times. I can't tell my family enough how much I love them and how important they are to me.

Things started to change for me when Charlie committed suicide. He was in pain every waking hour, as I remember. To watch your brother suffering and get more addicted to pain-killing drugs is terribly heart-wrenching. The hemophilia seemed harder on him than the other three bleeders. It got to be too much for him to handle, so he took his own life. I'm pretty sure Charlie would have been another victim of AIDS, had he lived. I miss him and think of him a lot, but I understand why he had to do it.

Donnie, the youngest child, and next to me in age, was diagnosed with AIDS while he was serving jail time in 1986. By the time he was released, the virus had started progressing. He died three years after being diagnosed. The last year of Donnie's life was the hardest thing I had ever faced. We saw him lose a lot of weight, develop skin infections, experience memory loss, and grow weaker as the days passed. I tried to give Donnie all the time that I could, that I should have given before he got sick. No one knows. I was sit ing at Donnie's side when he died. I'll never forget the smile of relief on his face as he left me. I love you, Donnie. I feel your spirit close to me a lot.

Donnie never really had the will or power to fight for his life. I believe mental attitude is such an important factor in fighting off AIDS. Donnie left behind a daughter and so many memories. Now, as we look to the future, we have two more brothers who were diagnosed with AIDS before Donnie was. But they have had that will to fight for life. They have been fighting this with every ounce of strength they can muster. Les seems to be losing the fight now, but he hasn't given up yet.

What an empty, lonely feeling thinking about losing a third brother, and knowing there's not a damned thing you can do about it. I will call him sometimes, just to hear his voice and tell him that I love him. He gets short-tempered sometimes, but I hope he understands that I have to do this. He has been to hell and back, like anyone with AIDS.

My other infected brother, Scott, is not as advanced as Les; but, how would you feel knowing that you will more than likely be the last boy alive dealing with AIDS along with the hemophilia. I sure as hell wouldn't want that burden.

My mom carries a burden that no one can imagine. She blames herself every day for giving the boys the hemophilia that, ultimately, led to the transmission of AIDS. They had no choice. They needed the blood products to control their hemophilia. They were robbed innocently, like thousands of bleeders; it was not a choice they could make.

It's very hard to be tough some days. Thank God for my family and close friends. They're always there for me.

Expressing myself and my feelings to other people hasn't been easy, but I've learned through this experience that I need to say it when I feel it, not shut it up inside, in that safe place. Our family has been through an awful lot of pain. We have stuck together and seen things through like most families do. But this family can't be denied the fact that we haven't had it one bit easy. We will stick together and see each other through all of this, but not without many scars, both emotional and physical, that will last us all a lifetime.

It's so important that they continue their research and find new drugs to treat, control, and, hopefully, cure AIDS so thousands of lives can be saved. They are trying to organize an AIDS support group locally. I hope people come forward and open up about this killer disease. I know my family will be involved.

In closing, I need to tell my family, especially Charlie, Donnie, Les, Scott, and Mom. I love you all very much.

RALPH

The human spirit is one of the most remarkable phenomena ever to grace this planet. It is at once resiliently stubborn in the face of extinction and wieldingly flexible to the pressure of survival. All around this world are stories of seemingly incredible hardship being endured, and at the same time fabulous technological breakthroughs being announced. As far as we know, we are the only species that can be proud of itself for the willful instinct not only to survive but to search relentlessly for an understanding of how and why we are.

My family has experienced both ends of the life spectrum. We are people who were facing near extinction but who benefited from a medical miracle that would all but eliminate our suffering, only to discover that this same miracle had brought with it an even more imminent danger. We feel a strong resentment toward the medical establishment for introducing AIDS into our family. Nevertheless, without their diligence, we might not have lived into the 1980s. And it is their current AIDS research that provides hope for all the remaining family members.

Since, in the early 1950s, I was an assumed hemophiliac child, an operation for my ruptured appendix would have been performed only if death was certain. Nasal tubes to pump the infection from inside me and intensive care treatment resulted in a "walled off" rupture, and surgery has been avoided to this day. As a maturing man in the late 1960s, I was classified 1A for the draft because there had been no instances of bleeds to warrant classification as a hemophiliac. I enlisted and was placed in the infantry. The 1970s were my own to grow and find a life with freedom from the feeling of oppression that resulted from the knowledge of constant pain felt by my mother and brothers. As the 1980s came to a close, I had come full circle and back to a feeling of medical uncertainty for my siblings. As a middle-aged man of the 1990s, my thoughts will be focused on facing AIDS, which has been introduced into my family by the medical treatments used to alleviate hemophilia. Not far removed are thoughts of our spouses and children and how they will endure the pain of sharing suffering with people they love.

The present members of my family more or less had time to learn about and adapt to the situation. Waiting in the wings is the next generation of our family, who will not have the luxury of time to adapt. We have invited them into our world, which includes not only a past of pain but a promise of potential hardship. Just as we have tried to leave that generation a better financial folder than we ourselves had, we need to leave them a better hospice folder as well.

Hospice care, both for Donnie and ourselves, was an unknown resource until the last few weeks of Donnie's life. The Hemophila Foundation had a counselor in St. Paul who tried to arrange a support group with us and point us to local hospice care. The distance necessary to travel to the Twin Cities on a regular basis doomed the attempt. My wife, Sharon, and I consulted with an independent hospice counselor here in our home town of Waseca; but she was unable to direct us to a hospice or support group in Mankato. We finally made contact with a brand-new agency, Prairie River Care Providers. The relief given to all of us was welcome indeed. From the very first visit by the providers to the end of Donnie's ordeal, it was evident that this service is a resource necessary for the comfort of the patient as well as the survival of the remaining family members. We will have an ongoing need for this service to comfort those who are both afflicted with and affected by the AIDS virus.

I am physically free of the discomfort of both hemophilia and AIDS. I never had to practice scooting down stairs on my bottom to avoid wear on ankles and knees, self-inject factorate, or avoid the vomiting of AZT. I do have a responsibility, as a member of this family, to participate in our struggle to achieve as near a normal living situation as possible. My self-imposed role is to do the things that others cannot, and to remind us that there is still so much to be thankful for and so much we can do for ourselves. Thinking about suffering doesn't make it go away; doing something about it does.

It is very easy to slip on blinders when pain and suffering land on someone's life. It is normal for people to focus absolutely on themselves during these periods. We usually return to normal when the hardship passes; but if it shows no sign of passing, we endure with the conviction, "that's how life is." Hardship becomes normal. Therefore, as long as all family members share the hardship as a normal part of their lives, any complaints heard within the family will fall on well-attuned and sympathetic ears.

The most important contribution that I make to our family is to balance our perception so we don't get lost in the negatives of the struggle. We have so much that is enjoyable and promising; we have memories of good times that far outnumber the bad. We have love for each other that many families should envy. We have produced a group of people steeped in the understanding of compassion so early in life that they don't consider it a special quality. For every negative we face, there is a compensating positive.

Mom feels tremendous guilt for the suffering of her many children and granchildren. Isn't a heavy load easier to carry with more to share the weight? If she questions whether we feel she was wrong to have had children or to have continued having them once she knew about the hemophilia, she can equally point to the many grandchildren we gave her when we all knew ourselves.

It has been urged that I not take the role of big brother to the entire family. The others, wanting to spare me exposure to the hardship and suffering, would set me and my own family free to get on with a "normal" life. But I am unable to let them go; I have no desire to belong to a family other than ours. I must, however, be willing to modify my contribution from time to time so that it has more value to the recipients, instead of being just what I think they require. I need to contribute what I have, as I need to share what they have.

We still have a big task ahead. There is more illness to face in the near future, but let's not forget the other facets of our lives. Our spouses and children, who are one step removed from the crisis, should not be forsaken during this present battle with AIDS. I think often of how frightening all this is for them. We must be careful to understand their fears and address their concerns. After all, we brought this to their lives, and we are responsible to teach them all the lessons we can. We must not let our present focus allow us to ignore their problems and uncertainties. It would be a great legacy to teach them to care for each other as we do.

Recent holidays especially have been thought of as "the last that we would all be together." Shouldn't we take advantage of them, then, as a chance to laugh and share good memories that will last a lifetime, no matter what its duration?

JEANETTE

My name is Jeanette Gimmer. I am the mother of three HIV/AIDS-infected hemophiliac sons. The fact that they have hemophilia is the important factor in this case. None of them is homosexual or an IV-drug user.

I will try to convey my feelings without going into too much autobiographical detail other than to say what I feel is necessary to try to convey to the readers, to help them understand, why anyone with even average intelligence would continue to bear children after learning that she was a carrier of a disease that can cause so much pain and suffering. I've always carried this terrible guilt complex because of the hemophilia, passing it to my boys. Ironically, I feel no malice toward my mother. Sometimes, when the boys look at me, I think maybe they'd like to punch me out. (And, sometimes, I wish they would.) But they've never (at least openly), criticized me for what's happened to them. I wonder how much criticism my daughters will get, as it's passed on down the line.

Of my eight children, I have three girls (in order of birth): Irma, Debbie, and Shari; and five boys (in order of birth): Charles, Ralph, Lawrence Scott, Leslie, and Donnie. The eldest son suffered all his life with hemophilia and became drug-dependent because of the pain in his joints, and took his own life at thirty-three years of age. I have no knowledge that he had AIDS.

Since this story is about sharing "death and dying," it has much to do with my history. I lost my mother, Irma, to nephritis when she was twenty-six. I was seven years old. My father, Chet, was an over-the-road truck driver and, although he did the best he could, he did not know what to do with a young daughter. I was placed in the care of various relatives, boarding care homes, and even with him and his second wife off and on.

Then, when I was barely sixteen, I gave birth to a beautiful daughter, Irma, and finally, I found what I had wanted and needed so desperately—someone who needed me, someone whom I could love and who would love me in return. I married her father, who was eight years my senior, and knew I would live happily ever after.

Since I had had virtually no contact with my mother's family since her death, I knew nothing about the hemophilia strain in her family. I knew Charlie definitely had something seriously wrong with him. Shortly after his birth, he almost bled to death from his circumcision. At that time, the doctor who treated him blamed the country hospital where he was born. Then, as he started walking and falling, biting his tongue or lip and bleeding nonstop, then bleeding into the joints, the doctors said he had pseudohemophilia. When Scott came along with similar problems, they finally suggested I contact my mother's family and ask some questions.

All I could learn from the remaining members of my mother's family was that she had three brothers who were "bleeders," two of whom had bled to death. I have since learned that I have at least one cousin who had a hemophiliac son. She wrote to me after the death of my youngest son, Donnie, who had AIDS, and said her son, too, had died from the disease.

The doctors in those days did not perform sterilization unless the life of the mother or child depended on it; as long as there was a chance that I would have girls or boys who did not inherit the disease and because I was so young, surgery was ruled out. When Leslie came along and had the same problem, the doctor suggested sterilization. However, his father refused to sign the permission slip.

I was married three times. My children as a group were with me alone more than with a father. We desperately loved and needed one another. Our feelings have not changed, even though they're grown and gone.

About six years ago, we found out that Lawrence, Leslie, and Donnie had contracted AIDS from the blood products they had received. At that time, the oldest of the three, Lawrence (Scott), was working on his doctorate. Leslie had just recently been married. The third one, the baby of my family, Donnie, had separate problems of his own, including pot and pills, burglary, domestic problems, and any other kind of problem that you can think of. He had to spend some time in prison.

When he came home, the onset of AIDS began. In prison, he was threatened and had to be kept under protection most of the time. He couldn't even complete his education. He lived with me until he died, almost two years ago. It was very, very difficult watching him go downhill, lose his hair, go through periods of severe aggression, depression, and weight loss. When Donnie was so sick, he didn't want anything to do with his friends when they would try to come and see him. When they did see how fast he was failing and how his appearance was changing, as well as his attitude, they seldom came back a second time. One very good friend, Ben, would come to read and do things for him. Donnie accepted Ben. They were childhood buddies, and Ben really took his death hard. Family, Donnie always loved. He still wanted them but the family had been turned off by his "antics" years before.

His sister, Shari, and his brother, Scott, tried. It was very difficult for them to see Donnie, to see how rapidly he was failing. He wouldn't eat. I coaxed him to eat all the time. He'd say, "O.K., Mommy, I'll try for you."

After he was on Prozac, his aggression stopped, but he was so dependent on me. I was working full time, but even when he was hospitalized, I'd go up there at noontime and try to get him to eat. He'd try, but he was so sick he just couldn't do it. His last few days, he came home and we set up a hospital bed there for him. He died at home.

Donnie's little girl, Cassie (who was only three years old when her father died), was so upset she had nightmares for months afterward. But she's accepted it now. When she goes by the cemetery, she waves at him and says, "Hi, dad." She goes out and puts flowers on the grave during holidays, but she still doesn't understand where her daddy is.

I thought Charlie's death was the most difficult thing I'd ever have to face. But it's the same every time it happens. Charlie left a son, Allan, who is not a hemophiliac and is as concerned about all this as the rest of us. Even though miles separate us, we all live on the same wavelength.

Now, my son Leslie is getting to the stage where Donnie was. He still can get up and around some, but he's very sick, and I know it won't be long before he's gone. It's going to be very difficult for Leslie's family. He has two stepdaughters who adore him. Even though I'm sure he's difficult to live with at times, it's going to be so hard on them. I worry about his wife. He has a beautiful wife. What is she going to do? As far as I know, she doesn't have the virus, but, if she does come down with it, what's going to become of those two little girls? If she doesn't, will another man want her? Les has fathered a daughter, Melanie. Her life is affected.

Scott is in much better shape, but we all know it's only a matter of time.

Irma has two daughters. Their children are all right, so far. Julie, the youngest, is expecting this month and I pray that the baby will be all right.

Debbie lives in California and has a son who is a hemophiliac; we all worry about him. So far, he's been all right as far as the AIDS goes, and they watch him quite closely.

I would gladly take the AIDS virus from all of my children, if only they could live. It's affecting all of us. Donnie and Leslie's grandmother is deeply hurt by all of this, and confused. She has never understood hemophilia.

I don't know what else I can say about death and dying, except that my problems began when I lost my mother. I have gone through all the stages of feeling, anger, and faith. I was so sure I could make Donnie well. It got to the point where he hated to see me come with a spoon in my hand, or a glass. But I knew God was with me through all that period. Now, what bothers me is that I no longer have that faith. I can no longer find my Lord to help me. Even though I know He's there, I'm angry because He's let this terrible thing happen, not only to me but to all of the innocent people in the country who are dying of AIDS. I do thank God, however, for the support of my family and my good friends throughout this ordeal. To my knowledge, we haven't been criticized that much, and definitely not ostracized.

I know this message sounds selfish. I refer to everything as me or mine, but as far as I'm concerned, these kids and I are one. Debbie, Leslie, Donnie, and Shari were one family; Scott, Charlie, Irma, and Ralph were another. I love all of them and the two families make for a lot of love.

I could say that this has brought us all closer together. Maybe in some ways it has, but we've always been a close-knit family, my children and I. I have always felt like the proverbial octopus; when I lost Charlie, I lost one of my tentacles. Two years, ago, I lost another one. Now I'm waiting to lose two more. I pray that I don't have to live long enough to lose them all. It isn't right that a parent should watch her children die. It should be the other way around. (And don't think I haven't considered suicide. But I wouldn't do that to my children.)

I know one way in which my lifestyle has changed. I used to be a meticulous housekeeper, full of ambition. Now, although I still work, my house goes to pot. I really don't care about it; it just exists. There doesn't seem to be any way that I can get motivated. I'm just always waiting for that other shoe to drop. I don't know where the answer lies.

Another problem I have to work through is my job. I work for the American Red Cross, and one of their primary functions is blood collection. For years, we had to depend on that blood. I have a deep, deep resentment even though I know that anybody who gave blood, who donated that blood, gave it in good faith. I know that when the boys received that blood, the Americ n Red Cross (or whoever gave it) was not aware that it was contaminated. Now, I have to work through the problem of trying to accept that. I don't work with that particular aspect in my job, if I can help it, because whenever I see the commercial on TV that represents the Red Cross Blood Program, I get very resentful and would like to throw something through the TV. But I know that I have to control it and overcome it. The blood that saved them all those years is the thing that's killing them.

Our hospital has finally come up with a support group. At least we're going to try to get one going. Maybe that'll help all of us, I don't know. Donnie's last month or so, he had wonderful support, and so did I, from Prairie River Health Care workers who came in and helped us. My daughter, Shari, spent a lot of time supporting Donnie and me. There were friends from St. Paul Ramsey and others Donnie had made in prison, religious people, who also came to see him. The minister of Our Savior's Church, Pastor Ortloff, was there for him. I wanted to have Donnie baptized. His dad would never let him be baptized, and Donnie didn't want to be baptized either, but he did tell the minister that he believed. The minister said that's all it took, that he didn't have to go through the ritual if he didn't want to.

Margie, the lady who lives with me, puts up with my moods and my snide remarks and tears, and through it all we try to keep a sense of humor, but I just. . . . There are so many people I need to thank who have been there for me. There are people from the hospital who came; they saw Donnie and helped with him. My close friends have also been there for us. I want to thank everybody.

One of my main regrets is that I could never sit down and really talk to Donnie or Scott or Les about this dying business. We all know it's there, but we don't know how to discuss it. The only thing Donnie ever said to me was a few months before he died. "Mom,

I'm only twenty-four years old, I'm too young too die." Right up to the last moment, I was determined that Donnie would live. I'm determined now that something could happen to keep me from losing these other two. I will continue to pray that they might make it, as long as I have even a shred of faith.

I have one friend, whose son is gay. He has had AIDS for a long, long time. He's on treatment, still holding his own, and still here with us. I also have learned of another old friend from school days. Her son has AIDS and so does his wife. She calls and writes to me for support. She can't understand it at all and she's having a very difficult time with it. I try to be there and be strong for her. I guess that's the best I can do. When I'm strong for others, it helps to keep my own strength up.

ACKNOWLEDGMENTS

Most of us will survive the experience with AIDS. With Donnie's loss still smarting, we are gathering our resources for the next deadly encounter. Among our allies, professional hospice care is the newest and potentially the most beneficial weapon we have. It may seem that our voices only mention this service in passing, but the impact of its comfort for even a few weeks has left a permanent impression. We have much to learn about this friend. Welcome to our side.

We would not have an opportunity to pass on these family voices if we did not have our spouses and children. They have spent their lives with us more or less silently, while we have expended most of our energies on our physical and related emotional struggles. This has taken a terrible toll on our families. A successful marriage is rare indeed, and in a case like ours, spouses can maintain a sense of normalcy for only so long before they are accused of "not understanding." Our children don't even have the chance to evacuate the battleground. For all the strange things we have brought to your lives, we humbly apologize.

A special thanks is in order to Sharon Hall for her hours of typing and editing this document. There would be no chance of hearing these voices without her help and concern.

Noticeably missing from these voices are Lawrence and Leslie. You won't hear complaining from them, because it is not the message they impart about their lives. They know better than all of us what lies ahead.

Lawrence has always conducted himself with a tomorrow in mind and there is no need to bother the family with too much of today's discomforts. He has published some thoughts, but they pertain to his profession of statistical analysis of behavior patterns for mentally disturbed patients.

Les loves his family and would not bring them discomfort with an issue that they cannot change. He has consistently made himself available to aid those of us in need, even though he seldom burdens the family when he is in need himself. He provides the connecting link between the four brothers. Their bond is a special thing, combining compassion, dignity, and pride.

Hospice care and related group support are such vital elements of the survival of families like ours. We have a big family. The diversity of its members has been a godsend for sharing this struggle. There is need for even more support and professional care than we have had access to. What about those little families of two to four members trying to cope? The people who reached out to us and provided soothing comfort to Jeanette cannot be thanked enough. The initial formation of a professional hospice group in our town will provide the opportunity for many people to survive the ordeal that is in danger of overwhelming us all.

Dr. Robert Buckingham's book is being published at a very important time in our family's life. It not only allows us a vehicle to voice our message, but codifies some principles that will aid our own survival. His lessons for hospice care will provide the framework to apply the compassion of healing without diminishing the dignity needed to face death. Dr. Buckingham's advice to the caregiver can be followed by family members, who are the primary care providers in some cases. Thank you.

Glossary of Medical Terms

Acetaminophen. A pain-relieving medication.

Acquired. Relating to a condition that is not inherited.

Acyclovir. An antiviral agent used to treat genital herpes.

Adenopathy. Enlargement or swelling of glands, especially the lymph nodes.

AIDS (Acquired Immunodeficiency Syndrome). A condition characterized by an impairment of the immune system, which leaves affected individuals susceptible to certain cancers and opportunistic infections. Currently a diagnosis is made based on the presence of one or more diseases or conditions as defined by the Centers for Disease Control (CDC). The CDC has proposed expanding the definition of AIDS to include all HIV-infected individuals with T-4 cell counts below 200 per measured unit of blood regardless of the presence of other diseases (see Helper T-cells).

179

Amphotericin-B. An antifungal drug given to patients with cryptoccocal infection, histoplasmosis, or severe candidiasis. Side effects of the drug include fever, chills, kidney toxicity, anorexia, and vomiting. (†)

Analgesic. An agent that reduces pain.

Anemia. A condition in which there is a lower than normal number of red blood cells. Typical symptoms include headaches, drowsiness, and general malaise. Patients with severe anemia may require blood transfusions.

Anorexia. Loss of appetite that may result in significant weight loss.

Antibody. A protein substance developed by the body, usually in response to stimulation by an antigen. Antibodies destroy or neutralize bacteria, viruses, or other harmful toxins.

Antigen. A foreign substance which, when introduced into the body, may trigger an immune response and the production of a specific antibody.

Antiviral Therapy. Treatment aimed at destroying a virus or suppressing its disease-causing action.

Aspergillosis. The presence of mold in the tissues and mucous membranes.

Attendant Care. Personal care and assistance with activities of daily living provided by a home health aide or homemaker.

AZT (Zidovudine or Retrovir). An antiviral drug approved by the Food and Drug Administration (FDA) in 1987, which has been proven effective in reducing the rate of opportunistic infections and increasing life expectency among individuals with HIV infection. (§)

Bactrim. An antibiotic given for treatment of Pneumocystis carinii pneumonia (PCP). Side effects of the drug include nausea, vomiting, and kidney toxicity (reversible). (‡)

Cachexia. A profound state of ill health and malnutrition.

Candidiasis. A fungal infection that involves the skin (dermatocandidiasis), mouth (oral thrush), esophagus (candida esophagitis), respiratory tract (bronchocandidiasis), and vagina (vaginitis). Candidiasis of the esophagus and respiratory tract is an indicator disease for AIDS.

Compassionate Use. A regulatory mechanism for releasing a new drug before it has been proven to be effective. The drug company is not allowed to charge patients for the drug. Special approval is required from the FDA for compassionate use of a drug.

Contagious. Referring to any infectious disease that can be transmitted casually from one person to another.

Cryptococcal Meningitis. A fungal infection that causes inflammation of the spinal cord or brain. Typical symptoms include headache, blurred vision, nausea, and confusion. Cryptococcal meningitis is one of the most frequent opportunistic infections in persons with AIDS.

Cryptococcoma. An infectious inflammatory lesion, in the brain, lung, or elsewhere.

Cryptosporidiosis. An infection caused by a parasite found in the intestines of animals which is transmitted to humans by direct contact with an infected animal or by ingestion of contaminated food or water. The infection causes chronic or intermittent severe diarrhea, and is accompanied by fever, weight loss, and enlarged lymph nodes.

Cyroprecipitate. A component of human blood that contains the compounds of blood clotting factors. It is condensed from whole blood or blood plasma for the purpose of supplementing the clotting deficiency of hemophiliacs.

Cytomegalovirus (CMV). A virus related to the herpes family. CMV infections may involve the eyes, central nervous system, lungs, and gastrointestinal tract. CMV can cause blindness in people with AIDS suffering from CMV-induced retinitis (see Retinitis). The disease cannot be cured. Patients are treated with intravenous DHPG (ganciclovir). If treatment is withdrawn, symptoms will recur.

Dapsone. An antibiotic given in combination with AZT or pentamidine for acute treatment and prevention of PCP. Side effects of the drug include anorexia and nausea and vomiting. (‡).

DDC (Dideoxycytidine). An antiviral drug currently under investigation study. Significant rises in CD-4 cell counts have been documented; however, approximately half of all patients receiving the drug have experienced reversible painful neuropathy. (§)

DDI (Dideoxyinosine). An antiviral drug currently under investigational study through an expanded access program designed to make the drug available to patients who cannot tolerate AZT. The drug is tolerated by most patients and is much less toxic than AZT. (§)

Dementia. Chronic deterioration of an individual's mental capacity, including memory, perception, judgment, and language.

DHPG (Ganciclovir). An antiviral agent used in the treatment of CMV retinitis. It must be given via an intravenous infusion and is available only on a compassionate use basis. (‡).

Diathesis. An inborn predisposition to certain medical conditions or abnormalities.

Dysthymic. Relating to mood disorder.

Electrolyte. A compound that, in solution, conducts electricity.

Encephalitis. Inflammation of the brain.

Epidemic. The occurrence of an infectious disease which attacks many people at the same time in the same geographical area.

Epstein-Barr Virus (EBV). A herpes-like virus that causes infectious mononucleosis. It has been associated with Burkitt's lymphoma and hairy leukoplakia (see Lymphoma and Hairy Leukoplakia).

Factorate. The commonly used name of the manufactured antihemophiliate administered to induce clotting of human blood. In at least one case, Antihemophiliate Factorate is part of a trade name.

Factor Eight. One of ten blood-clotting components the deficiency of which results in a genetic condition labeled as hemophilia A or classic hemophilia (also noted as factor 8 or factor viii).

Fluconazole. An antfungal drug given for cryptococcal meningitis and candidias. Side effects of the drug include nausea and vomiting. (‡)

Gastrointestinal. Relating to the stomach and intestines.

Genitourinary. Relating to the organs of reproduction and urination.

Hairy Leukoplakia. A whitish, slightly raised lesion found on the side of the tongue which has been associated with the Epstein-Barr Virus infection.

Health Care Financing Administration (HCFA) The federal agency responsible for administering the Medicare and Medicaid programs.

Helper T-cells (T4, CD4, T-cells). A laboratory value that is frequently used to assess the status of an HIV-infected patient. T-cells help fight off infection and are normally present at 1,000 per measured unit of blood.

Hemophilia. A hereditary, sex-linked disease limited to males and characterized by impaired clotting of the blood, resulting in a strong tendency to bleed. Treatment is aimed at raising the level of clotting factor eight, which is found in fresh whole blood or blood plasma (se Factor Eight).

Herpes Simplex Virus I (HSV I). A virus that causes cold sores or fever blisters on the mouth, throat, or eyes and can be transmitted to the genital area. The latent virus can be reactivated by stress, other infections, or a compromised immune status.

Herpes Simplex Virus II (HSV II). A virus that cause painful sores of the anus or genitals. It may lie dormant in nerve tissue and can be reactivated to produce the sores.

Herpes Variacella Zoster Virus (HVZ). The reactivation of the varicella virus in adults, which is the same virus that causes chicken pox as a child. Herpes zoster, also known as shingles, is characterized by very painful blisters on the skin following nerve pathways.

Histoplasmosis. A disease contracted from mold and manifested by an inflammation of the lungs with clinical features similar to those of tuberculosis.

HIV (Human Immunodeficiency Virus). The virus that causes AIDS. HIV is transmitted by three routes: sexual contact; parenteral exposure to infected blood (through blood transfusions or sharing of needles); and perinatal contact, from an infected mother to her infant.

HIV Seronegative. Showing no trace of HIV infection.

HIV Seropositive. Showing antibodies as the result of prior infection with HIV.

Immune Deficiency. A breakdown in an individual's immune system, making the individual susceptible to diseases that he or she would not ordinarily develop.

Intravenous Drugs. Drugs injected by needle directly into a vein.

Kaposi's Sarcoma. A rare malignant skin tumor that occurs in some people with AIDS. Kaposi's sarcoma usually appears as purplish lesions on the skin but may also occur in the gastrointestinal tract, lymphatic system, lungs, or liver.

Leukoencephalopathy. A disease of the brain tissue that may occur in people with suppressed immune systems.

Leukopenia. A lower than normal level of circulating white blood cells. It may predispose an individual to infections when the count is very low.

Lymphoma. A general term referring to a number of malignancies in which various cells in the body's lymphatic system have proliferated out of control. Lymphomas frequently seen in people with AIDS include non-Hodgkins lymphomas and Kaposi's sarcoma.

Medicaid. A state and federally funded, state-administered health insurance program for low-income persons.

Medicare. The federal health insurance program for the elderly, the permanently disabled, and individuals with end-stage kidney disease.

Mycobacterium Avium Intracellulare (MAI). A bacterial infection that can involve the gastrointestinal tract, lungs, bone marrow, or liver. MAI infections are common opportunistic infections of terminally ill AIDS patients. Symptoms may include fatigue, fever, night sweats, weight loss, and diarrhea.

Neutropenia. An abnromally low neutrophil (white blood cell) count, which can leave a patient susceptible to bacterial and fungal infections.

Opportunistic Infection. An infection with any organisms that occurs when the host's immune system is compromised.

Oncology. A brand of medicine that deals with tumors.

Oropharynx. The area of the mouth and upper windpipe.

Palliative. Referring to treatment aimed at offering relief not cure.

Pandemic. An epidemic disease that is occuring at the same time in many different parts of the world.

Papovavirus. A virus that replicates in nuclei of infected cells, which may produce tumors.

Pathogen. Any microorganism or virus that can cause disease.

Pentamidine. An FDA-approved drug for the treatment or prevention of PCP. The drug is given either intravenously or through inhalation, and is recommended for patients who have had at least one episode of PCP or who have CD4-cell counts below 200. (§)

Peripheral Neuropathy. Damage to the nerves in the feet, hands, or legs. Symptoms may include pain, numbness, and a tingling sensation.

Pneumocystis Carinii Pneumonia (PCP). A severe, life-threatening lung infection found in 80 percent of all people with AIDS at some time during the course of their illness.

Prophylaxis. Treatment aimed at preserving health and preventing the spread of disease.

Retinitis. Inflammation of the retina. CMV-induced retinitis is a common opportunistic infection in people with AIDS.

Somatic. Relating to the body.

Syndrome A group of symptoms that characterize a specific disease or condition.

Thrush. See Candidiasis.

Toxoplasmosis. A common opportunistic infection and a leading cause of encephalitis in persons with HIV infection. It may also involve the heart, lung, adrenal glands, pancreas, and testes.

Vaccine. A substance containing components of an infectious organism which is given to an individual for the purpose of establishing resistance to an infectious disease. To date, there is no vaccine available to protect against HIV.

Code for Medications:

† Not usually given to hospice patients.

‡ Given to hospice patients.

§ Given initially to hospice patients, then gradually discontinued.

Note: This glossary is intended as a guide only. Each hospice organization may determine their own terms and guidelines.

Select Bibliography

AIDS Homecare and Hospice in San Francisco: A Model for Compassionate Care. Special Issue: AIDS. Denver, Colorado, 1986.

Alger I. "Interactive Videodiscs: Suicide and Chronic Mental Illness." *Hospital Community Psychiatry* 40, no. 6 (June 1989): 582–83.

Andersen, Heather, and Penny MacElveen-Hoehn. "Gay Clients with AIDS: New Challenges for Hospice Programs." *Hospice Journal* 4 (1988).

Bialer, P. A., and J. J. Wallack. "Mixed Factitious Disorder Presenting as AIDS." *Hospice Community Psychiatry* (May 1990).

Buckingham and Saunders. "Suicidal AIDS Patients: When the Depression Turns Deadly." *Nursing* 18, no. 7 (July 1988): 59–64.

Clark et al. "Hospice Care: A Model for Caring for the Person with AIDS." *Nurses Clin. North Am.* 23, no. 4 (December 1988): 851–62.

Cohen. "Biopsychosocial Approach to the Human Immunodeficiency Virus Epidemic." *General Hospital Psychiatry* (March 12, 1990): 98–123.

189

Derek, Humphry. "The Case for Rational Suicide." *Euthanasia Review* 1 (Fall 1986).

Doebbert et al. "AIDS and Suicide in California." *Journal of the American Medical Association* 260, no. 13 (October 7): 1881.

Fishman et al. "Suicidal Ideation and HIV Testing." *Journal of the American Medical Association* (February 2, 1990): 679–82.

Fraser et al. "AIDS Homecare and Hospice in San Francisco: A Model for Compassionate Care." *Journal of Palliative Care* 4 (December 1988).

Frierson and Lippmann. "Suicide and AIDS." *Psychosomatics* 29, no. 2 (Spring 1988): 226–31.

Glass. "AIDS and Suicide." *Journal of the American Medical Association* 259, no. 9 (March 4, 1988): 1369–70.

Hsu et al. "Increased Risk of Suicide in Persons with AIDS." *Journal of the American Medical Association* 259, no. 9 (March 4, 1988): 1333–37.

Jimenez, M. A., and D. R. Jimenez. "Training Volunteer Caregivers of Person with AIDS." *Social Work Health Care* 14, no. 3 (1990): 73–85.

Karlinsky et al. "Suicide Attempts and Resuscitation Dilemmas." *General Hospital Psychiatry* 10, no. 6 (November 1988).

McKegney and O'Dowd. "AIDS Patients Compared with Others Seen in Psychiatric Consultation." *General Hospital Psychiatry* (January 12, 1990): 50–55.

Marzuk. "AIDS Patients Are at Increased Risk for Suicide." *American Family Physician* 38, no. 3 (September 1988): 243.

Neppe et al. "Factitious AIDS." *Psychosomatics* 30 (Summer 1989): 702–707.

Nyamathi and Van Servellen. "Maladaptive Coping in the Critically Ill Population with Acquired Immunodeficiency Syndrome: Nursing Assessment and Treatment." *Heart Lung* 18, no. 2 (March 1989): 113–20.

Papathomopoulos, Evangelos. "Intentional Infection with the AIDS Virus as a Means of Suicide." *Counseling Psychology Quarterly* 2, no. 1: 79–81.

"The Risk of Suicide in Persons with AIDS." *Journal of the American Medical Association* 260, no. 1 (July 1, 1988): 29–30.

Schmitt, Laurent, et al. "Suicide and AIDS." *Psychologie Médicale* 21, no. 4 (March 1989).

Seymour, J. "Delusions of Having AIDS." *Psychiatry* 146, no. 4 (April 1989): 556.

Stephany T. "AIDS and the Home Nurse." *Home Health Nurse* 8, no. 2 (March–April 1990). 11–12.

Vomvouras. "Psychiatric Manifestations of AIDS Spectrum Disorders." *South. Med. J.* 82, no. 3 (March 1989): 352–57.